THE HEAD AND NECK

TO MY ANATOMY TEACHERS —

*MRS J. MOSELEY, PROFESSOR R.J. LAST,
DR F. STANSFIELD* AND THE
MANY STUDENTS OF THE SCHOOLS OF
MEDICINE IN UNIVERSITY COLLEGE
LONDON, UNIVERSITY OF OTTAWA,
CANADA, AND UNIVERSITY OF
CALIFORNIA, IRVINE

CLINICAL ANATOMY IN ACTION   VOLUME 2

THE HEAD AND NECK

John Pegington FRCS(Eng)

Senior Lecturer, Department of Anatomy, and Honorary
Senior Lecturer, Department of Surgery, University College
London; Examiner Part 1, FRCS(Ed); Past Associate
Professor, Anatomy Department, Faculty of Health Sciences,
Ottawa, Canada ; S.A. Courtauld Professor, Middlesex
Hospital

Illustrations by
Melody Crocker DFA(Lond) PGCE

Photographic preparation by
Mike Gilbert

CHURCHILL LIVINGSTONE
EDINBURGH LONDON MELBOURNE AND NEW YORK 1986

CHURCHILL LIVINGSTONE
Medical Division of Longman Group UK Limited

Distributed in the United States of America by Churchill
Livingstone Inc., 1560 Broadway, New York, N.Y. 10036, and
by associated companies, branches and representatives
throughout the world.

© Longman Group UK Limited 1986

First published 1986

ISBN 0 443 02869 0

British Library Cataloguing in Publication Data
Pegington, John
   Clinical anatomy in action.
   Vol. 2, The head and neck
   1. Anatomy, Human
   I. Title
   611   QM23.2

Library of Congress Cataloging in Publication Data
Pegington, John.
   Clinical anatomy in action.
   Includes indexes.
   Contents: v. 1. The vertebral column and limbs —
v. 2. [without special title]
      1. Anatomy, Human — Collected works. 2. Anatomy,
Pathological — Collected works. 3. Anatomy, Surgical
and topographical — Collected works. I. Title.
[DNLM: 1. Anatomy. QS 4 P375c]
QM5.P43   1985   611   84-9470

Printed and bound in Great Britain by
William Clowes Limited, Beccles and London

PREFACE

In writing this book, I assume that the reader has at some time studied the subject of human anatomy. Anatomical knowledge, however, tends to fade during the years of clinical work when it is often most needed. This text is *not* meant to replace the 'standard' textbooks, but rather to be a supplementary book designed to help recall important areas of anatomy in a palatable format. The title *Clinical Anatomy in Action* is meant to emphasise to the senior medical student that what he has learned is useful in clinical situations. I have tried to do this by using case studies. I hope that the selection of case histories will stimulate the student to think more deeply about the use of anatomy in everyday clinical work. The cases reflect the sort of problems commonly encountered during medical training, although I have also included one or two more uncommon conditions. The case studies are printed in contrasting type, and can easily be identified. If the student wishes, therefore, he can read the entire case at once, along with the chapter, or leave it out.

Most clinical anatomy books do not, in my opinion, give enough space to an explanation of radiographs and other imaging techniques. I have tried to redress such a deficiency in this book. I have left most of the radiographs *without labels*; this is how they will present for inspection in real-life situations. I have, however, tried to explain how to read them in the text. Learning to interpret radiographs requires active participation of the student, and I hope that he will try to label the radiographs himself and ask help from his tutors when needed. I have used this volume to introduce the student to the study of computed tomography and magnetic resonance imaging. Scans have been introduced into the text and into the case histories. The student should be familiar with all the modern imaging methods, and well informed about their place in diagnosis. The remarkable detail that can be achieved in many imaging techniques makes a knowledge of anatomy even more essential to the physician of today. In the foreseeable future, radiographs, CT scans and MRI scans will be available to the physician in his consulting room on a TV monitor.

The anatomy of the head and neck covers the territory of several medical specialties. The anatomy is of interest to the accident surgeon, the ophthalmologist, the ENT surgeon, the plastic surgeon, the general surgeon and to those concerned with the treatment of malignant conditions of the region. Many aspects of head and neck anatomy will therefore be required during the clinical years of training. Many find the region particularly difficult, but I can assure the student that a careful study of the head and neck will produce a rich reward.

I must assume that the reader actually wishes to review the subject of human anatomy. It is possible of course to practice medicine with only a scanty anatomical knowledge, but this can be neither stimulating nor rewarding. It is unfortunate that some students will have already been put off the subject during the first contact in medical school. I am sorry to report that I also suffered this fate, but was happily rescued during early surgical training. The problem is not new; Humphry noted it as early as 1861 in his book *The Human Foot and the Human Hand*. 'It must be confessed', he wrote, 'that we teachers of Anatomy are somewhat to blame. We are too prone, in our lectures and examinations, to dwell upon bare details, without enlivening these details with the many bright features of interest with which they are naturally invested.' I hope, in some small way, that *Clinical Anatomy in Action* will provide medical students, young graduates, and paramedical students, with a readable insight into some important aspects of anatomy. I further hope that for some it will start a life-long interest in the subject.

Special thanks are due to Miss Melody Crocker, a graduate of the Slade School of Fine Art and an experienced medical illustrator, for her skill and patience in preparing the artwork for these books. I am deeply indebted to Mr Mike Gilbert of the Photography Unit in the Department of Anatomy at University College London for the high quality of his work during preparation of the photographs. I thank Dr David Edwards, Head of the Department of Radiology at University College London, for his encouragement and advice, and for the many radiographs and CT scans. I must extend these thanks to Mr Liam Flood, Dr Peter Hamlyn, Dr David Gartry, Professor W. Ian McDonald, Dr J. Pennock and Dr B. M. Thomas for providing radiographs, CT and MRI scans. I am also very grateful to Mrs Sue Pryer and Dr David Gartry for reading the proofs.

Finally, I thank the Publishers, Churchill Livingstone, for asking me to write a book on clinical anatomy, and members of the publishing staff, for their enthusiasm, help and patience during its preparation.

London, 1986   J. P.

CONTENTS

PART ONE

The Cranium

1

THE BONES OF THE CRANIUM

CASES 1, 2 AND 3

Tom Talbott, Dick Duster, and Harry Harper were workers at a desert oil rig. A landrover carrying the three men hit a rock and overturned while they were returning to base from a field trip. Following the accident, Tom and Dick were unconscious, but Harry was able to call for help on the radio. All three men were rescued and examined within 30 minutes at the medical centre.

The attending physician first assessed the level of consciousness in all three patients. He used the Glascow coma scale to document the levels of consciousness (Table 1.1). Baseline observations of this sort form an important first step in the assessment of every head injury case, and give a good initial indication of the amount of brain damage. The score ranges from 3 to 15 when the full scale is used. Tom was deeply unconscious, and fresh blood was found running from his right ear. He did not open his eyes spontaneously or as a result of a painful stimulus. He therefore scored 1

Table 1.1 The Glascow coma scale

Function tested	Response	Score
1. Eye opening	Spontaneous	4
	To speech	3
	To pain	2
	None	1
2. Best verbal response	Oriented	5
	Confused conversation	4
	Inappropriate words	3
	Incomprehensible sounds	2
	None	1
3. Best motor response	Obeys commands	6
	Localises	5
	Flexes normally	4
	Flexes abnormally	3
	Extends	2
	None	1

on the scale for the ability to open the eyes. He made occasional incomprehensible sounds and was therefore scored as 2 on the verbal response scale. He did not move, apart from irregular extension movements of the limbs. The best motor response was therefore scored as 2. The total score was 5. While doing this quick assessment, the attendant had recorded the pulse, blood pressure, and respiration rate. His blood pressure was low (110/60), and his pulse rate rapid and feeble (120/min). Apart from examination of the head injury, the physician also quickly examined Tom's neck, thorax, abdomen, pelvis and limbs. He found a large bruise across the left upper abdominal wall and lower chest. Such a bruise, situated over the spleen, could indicate an injury sufficient to cause a rupture of this organ. A needle was therefore inserted into the peritoneal cavity in each of the four quadrants. Fresh blood was aspirated from the upper left tap, thus confirming intra-abdominal trauma and haemorrhage. An intravenous infusion had been started by the attendant. While these investigations were being carried out, the nurse took radiographs of the skull. It was clear that Tom had two conditions, a serious head injury and intra-abdominal trauma: multiple system involvement is not uncommon in severe injury.

Dick had regained consciousness by the time he was seen in the medical centre. His eye opening was spontaneous (4), his verbal response was confused (4), but he obeyed commands (6). His total score was 14 on the Glascow scale. He had a laceration over the right temporal region, but had no other obvious injuries. Radiographs were taken of his skull.

Harry was also conscious, and although he could not remember the accident itself, he remembered driving the landrover. He had thus suffered concussion accompanied by amnesia. He had a large bruise over the right frontal bone, but other—wise seemed to be in fairly good shape.

The physician and his team had made rapid initial assessments of the conditions of Tom, Dick and Harry. As you learn more about the head in this and the next few chapters, you will be able to follow and understand the progress of these and other cases.

THE VAULT OF THE SKULL

1. The bones of the vault

The calvaria, or bony vault of the cranium, consists of the frontal bone, paired parietal bones, and the occipital bone. On each side it is completed by the greater wings of the sphenoid and the squamous part of the temporal bone (Figs. 1.1, 1.5). The frontal bone forms the forehead, and it articulates behind with the two parietal bones at the coronal suture. The parietal bones themselves articulate in the midline at the sagittal suture. The Y-shaped junction made by the coronal and sagittal sutures is called the 'bregma' (Fig. 1.2). The most convex parts of the parietal bones are the parietal tubera, and the distance between them is the widest part of the skull. A parietal foramen is often found on each side of the sagittal suture, and when present, transmits a small emissary vein. The parietal bones articulate behind with the occipital bone at the lambdoid suture. The Y-shaped junction between the sagittal and lambdoid suture is called the 'lambda' (Fig. 1.3). Occasionally accessory sutural bones are found in the lambdoid suture. The occipital bone presents an external occipital protuberance half way between the lambda and the foramen magnum, and the most prominent part of this protuberance is the inion (Fig. 1.4). A superior nuchal line can be traced from this bony elevation on either side, and marks the origin of the trapezius and the insertion of the sternocleidomastoid. The highest nuchal line is found above the superior nuchal line and gives attachment to the occipital belly of occipitofrontalis.

The bones making up the rest of the calvaria are best seen on a lateral view of the skull (Fig. 1.5). The frontal bone articulates with the zygomatic bone in the lateral orbital margin at the zygomaticofrontal suture. Behind this, wedged between frontal, parietal, and squamous temporal bones is the greater wing of the sphenoid. The sutures involved in these articulates form an H-shape on the side of the skull, and this junction is called the

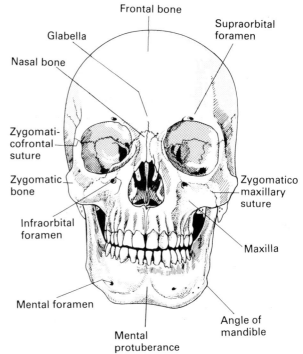

Fig. 1.1 The front of the skull

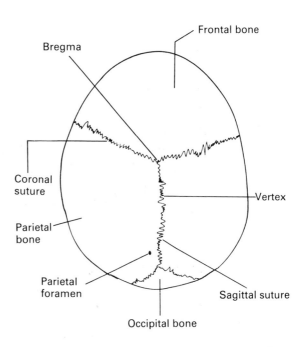

Fig. 1.2 The top of the skull

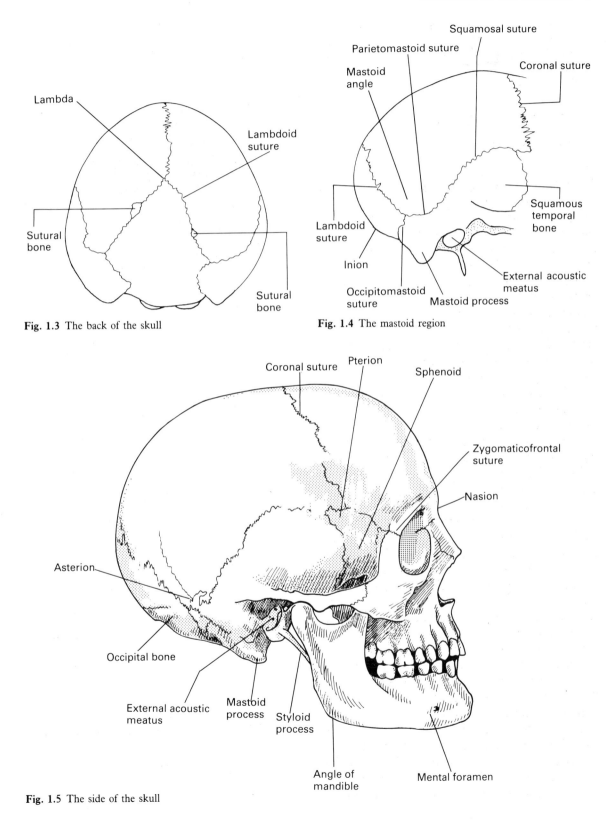

Fig. 1.3 The back of the skull

Fig. 1.4 The mastoid region

Fig. 1.5 The side of the skull

'pterion'. Curved superior and inferior temporal lines may be found high on the lateral surface of the skull arching back over both frontal and parietal bones. The superior line may be traced down as far as the mastoid region where it curves above the external acoustic meatus as the supramastoid crest. The temporalis muscle attaches to the skull below the inferior temporal line, and the strong fascia covering the muscle is attached to the superior temporal line. The squamous part of the temporal bone is fan-shaped, and articulates with the parietal bone at the squamosal suture, the bone often overlapping the parietal bone at this articulation. Behind the squamous temporal bone the parietal bone forms a narrow mastoid angle, and the lambdoid suture traced downwards to this angle becomes continuous with the occipitomastoid suture (Fig. 1.4). The mastoid process and the external acoustic meatus are described in Chapter 4.

The flat bones of the vault of the skull consist of outer and inner layers (tables) of compact bone separated by an intermediate layer of cancellous bone called the 'diploë'. The inner layer of bone is thinner than the outer, and may be fractured from a blow to the skull without evidence of injury to the outer table. Fractures of the calvaria are slow to heal, there being little capacity for regeneration associated with the periosteum in this region. Fractures in the temporal region heal better than elsewhere, possibly because of the rich blood supply to the bones from adjacent temporal arteries.

2. Blood supply and venous drainage of the calvaria

The arterial supply to the bones of the calvaria comes from arteries both outside and inside the skull. Temporal arteries, for example, send nutrient branches into the bones at the sides of the skull. Much of the supply, however, comes from meningeal arteries inside the cranial cavity. The supply is plentiful, because the diploë is a site for erythropoiesis. Meningeal arteries in the anterior cranial fossa come from ethmoidal and ophthalmic arteries. Occasionally, branches of the sphenopalatine arteries ascend from the nose to the fossa through the cribriform plate of the ethmoid to add to this supply. Meningeal branches of the internal carotid artery supply bone in the base of the middle cranial fossa, and an accessory meningeal branch of the maxillary artery often ascends through the foramen ovale to assist this supply. The largest of the meningeal arteries, however, is the middle meningeal artery. It is responsible for supplying the meninges above the tentorium cerebelli, and much of the bone of the vault. The middle meningeal artery, a branch of the maxillary artery, ascends through the foramen spinosum. It divides a short distance above the foramen into frontal and parietal branches. The surface marking of its main trunk lies approximately one thumb breadth behind the zygomatic process of the frontal bone, and two finger breadths above the zygomatic arch itself. Here it divides. The frontal branch curves upwards deep to the pterion, and then curls back in a broad curve a short distance behind the coronal suture. Occasionally the artery may run through a canal in the bone itself. The parietal branch of the artery passes horizontally to the back of the skull above the tentorium. It should be appreciated that there is variation in the pattern of the middle meningeal artery, and it does not always follow the course outlined. The ophthalmic artery, for example, may have an aberrant origin from the middle meningeal artery. The middle meningeal artery is distributed widely, and anastomoses with its fellow of the opposite side and with other meningeal vessels. Vertebral and occipital arteries provide meningeal branches to the posterior cranial fossa.

Blood is drained from the calvaria by diploic veins. These form large channels within the bone, and anastomose freely with each other. Four major vessels are described on each side: frontal, anterior temporal, posterior temporal, and occipital diploic veins. The veins drain both into venous sinuses inside the skull and into veins on the outside of the skull. The frontal diploic vein communicates with the superior sagittal sinus internally, and empties by a vessel which leaves through a hole in the skull at the supraorbital notch to empty into the supraorbital vein. The anterior temporal veins drain both into the sphenoparietal sinus inside the cranial cavity and into temporal veins on the outside. The posterior temporal vein drains into the transverse sinus and into the mastoid emissary vein.

The occipital diploic vein empties externally into the occipital veins and internally into the transverse sinus. Occasionally the veins become enlarged, and present a startling picture on a lateral radiograph of the skull. Such enlargement usually has no clinical significance.

THE INTERIOR OF THE SKULL

The student should study this section with the aid of a skull. Inside the cranial cavity, the base of the skull presents three cranial fossae. These are described as anterior, middle and posterior fossae (Fig. 1.6).

1. The anterior cranial fossa

Much of the floor of the anterior cranial fossa consists of the orbital plates of the frontal bone. Wedged between these two plates in the midline is the cribriform plate of the ethmoid. The crista galli projects upwards from the cribriform plate, and is continuous below with the perpendicular plate of the ethmoid in the nasal septum. The olfactory bulbs lie in contact with the cribriform plates, and about 15–20 olfactory nerve fibres ascend through the holes in the plate to enter the lower surface of the bulbs. Meningeal twigs from vessels in the nose may also travel through the cribriform plate and enter the anterior cranial fossa. Anterior ethmoidal nerves and vessels from the

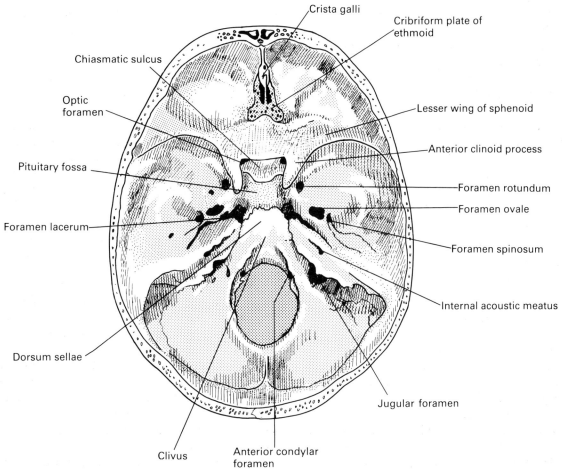

Fig. 1.6 The interior of the skull

orbit also reach the anterior cranial fossa through an anterior ethmoidal foramen situated between the ethmoid and frontal bones. Their course in the anterior cranial fossa, however, is brief, for they descend through a nasal slit on the side of the crista galli and reach the nose. While in the anterior cranial fossa the anterior ethmoidal nerve supplies sensory branches to the dura: stimulation of the dura in the floor of the fossa produces pain in the homolateral eye. In front of the crista galli is a small depression called the 'foramen caecum'. Although usually a blind pit, it sometimes conducts a small vein to the nose. A midline ridge, the frontal crest, may be traced forwards from the foramen caecum.

The posterior edge of the anterior cranial fossa is formed by the sphenoid bone. A ridge called the 'jugum sphenoidale' may be found on the body of this bone, below which is the chiasmatic sulcus. Extending laterally on either side from the jugum are the lesser wings of the sphenoid. At its origin, each lesser wing bears an anterior clinoid process which points back towards the middle cranial fossa.

The lower parts of the frontal lobes of the brain lie in the anterior cranial fossa, and some gyri leave depressions on the orbital plates. The lesser wings insinuate themselves in the stem of the lateral sulcus of the brain.

2. The middle cranial fossa

The floor of the middle cranial fossa is made up of the sphenoid and temporal bones. The sella turcica (Turkish saddle) of the sphenoid occupies the mid-part of the fossa. The concavity in the sella is the pituitary or hypophyseal fossa, and a small elevation, the tuberculum sellae, will be found on the front wall of the fossa. In front of the tuberculum is the chiasmatic sulcus, which leads on either side to an optic canal. Although named the 'chiasmatic sulcus', the optic chiasma is not always lodged in the groove, for the chiasma usually lies a little further back in the sella. The anterior clinoid processes overlap the pituitary fossa to some extent. Posteriorly, the fossa is limited by a sharp, horizontal ridge of bone called the 'dorsum sellae' which bears a posterior clinoid process on either side. (The clinoids were so named

because they were likened to the posts of a four-poster bed.) Very rarely, a patent craniopharyngeal canal, a remnant of embryological development, may be found in the depths of the fossa.

The middle cranial fossa is deep on each side of the sella turcica, and houses a temporal lobe of the brain. Here, the fossa is formed by the greater wing of the sphenoid and the temporal bone. The sphenoid bone has several foramina. Between the overhanging edge of the lesser wing and the greater wing is the superior orbital fissure, a slit which transmits many nerves and vessels to the orbit. Below this fissure is the foramen rotundum, leading forwards to the pterygopalatine fossa, and transmitting the maxillary nerve. Posterolateral to the foramen rotundum is the foramen ovale, and this transmits the mandibular division of the 5th nerve together with a secretomotor nerve for the parotid gland, and several small arteries and veins. Behind the foramen ovale is the foramen spinosum. The middle meningeal vessels ascend through this hole, together with the meningeal branch of the mandibular nerve (nervus spinosus). The grooves made by the middle meningeal vessels may be traced on the inner table of the skull from the foramen spinosum. The groove for the frontal branch curls upwards towards the pterion then curves backwards. Occasionally the vessels run in a bony tunnel in the bone. The groove for the parietal branch passes horizontally backwards across the squamous part of the temporal bone towards the occiput. Accessory foramina are occasionally found in the sphenoid bone. A foramen of Vesalius is sometimes found anteromedial to the foramen ovale, and when present transmits emissary veins. Behind the foramen ovale, between it and the foramen spinosum, a foramen innominatum will occasionally be found, and the meningeal branch of the mandibular nerve then uses this route to get to the middle cranial fossa.

Both squamous and petrous parts of the temporal bone are found in the middle cranial fossa. The petrous part of the temporal bone is in the form of a three-sided pyramid lying on its side. The apex points medially and forward towards the body of the sphenoid, while the base points laterally towards the external ear. The sharp upper edge extending from apex to base forms the boundary between the middle and posterior cranial fossae. From this so-called 'petrous ridge', the anterior slope of the bone extends into the middle cranial fossa and the posterior slope into the posterior fossa. The apex of the petrous temporal bone does not meet the sphenoid. A gap remains between the two bones called the 'foramen lacerum'. In life, this is filled with fibrocartilage, although occasional emissary veins may pass through it. On the anterior slope of the petrous temporal bone, near to the middle of the petrous ridge, is the arcuate eminence, an elevation which overlies the anterior semicircular canal. Further laterally the petrous temporal bone is thin, and forms the roof of the middle ear. This thin plate is called the 'tegmen tympani'. Two small slits can be found on the anterior slope for petrosal nerves. The larger of the two is for the greater petrosal nerve, and the smaller medial slit is for the lesser petrosal nerve. On the anterior slope, at the apex of the petrous temporal bone, is a hollow called the 'trigeminal impression' which is occupied in life by the large trigeminal ganglion. Hidden below the apex of the petrous temporal bone, and overlying the foramen lacerum, is the anterior end of the carotid canal. The internal carotid artery enters the skull through this canal and then travels along the side of the body of the sphenoid in a carotid groove in the bone. The groove can be traced upwards along the body of the sphenoid to the medial side of the anterior clinoid process. Occasionally a middle clinoid process is found on the edge of the sella and may fuse with the anterior clinoid process to form a foramen for the carotid artery.

CASE 4

Dotty Dobson, a 50-year-old schoolteacher, noticed vision worsening in both eyes over a period of 6 months. She also complained of visual hallucinations during which she thought that she saw faces. She was given leave of absence from her job and was referred to a psychiatrist. After initial psychological appraisal, however, he decided to investigate the possibility of an intracranial lesion close to the pituitary fossa as a cause of her symptoms.

3. The posterior cranial fossa

The mid-part of the floor of the posterior cranial fossa is formed in front by the body of the sphenoid. This presents a sloping surface from the dorsum sellae above to the occipital bone below. The combined slope of sphenoid and occipital bones from dorsum sellae to foramen magnum is called the 'clivus'. On each side, the anterior wall of the posterior cranial fossa is formed by the posterior slope of the petrous temporal bone, the most prominent feature of which is the internal acoustic meatus. This leads into a canal about 10 mm long. The lateral end of the canal is called the 'fundus', and here there are a number of foramina in the bone for transmission of the facial and vestibulocochlear nerves. Just above the internal acoustic meatus is a small depression called the 'subarcuate fossa', seen most clearly in the skull of a young child. Just lateral to the fossa is a small slit in the bone leading to the aqueduct of the vestibule. The endolymphatic duct occupies this aqueduct, and its dilated end, the endolymphatic sac, lies in the slit just deep to the dura. If a perpendicular is dropped from the internal acoustic meatus, a pyramidal notch will be located in the lower edge of the petrous temporal bone. This notch houses the glossopharyngeal nerve, and the aqueduct of the cochlea opens into its depths. The notched edge of the petrous temporal bone with the jugular notch of the occipital bone form the jugular foramen, a large irregular opening in the posterior cranial fossa. Apart from transmitting the 9th, 10th and 11th cranial nerves, it also transmits venous sinuses. The course of these sinuses in the posterior cranial fossa is marked by deep grooves in both temporal and occipital bones. The groove for the superior sagittal sinus is usually continuous with a groove for the right transverse sinus. This can be traced into a deep S-shaped groove in the mastoid part of the temporal bone. This houses the sigmoid sinus, and can be traced to the posterior part of the jugular foramen. A groove made by the superior petrosal sinus will be found on the upper edge of the petrous ridge, and it leads to the sigmoid groove. On the lower edge of the petrous temporal bone is a groove for the inferior petrosal sinus, and this leads to the front of the jugular foramen.

Posteriorly, the occipital bone has an internal occipital protuberance in the midline, and an internal occipital crest leading from here to the foramen magnum. The anterior condylar or hypoglossal canals are partly hidden in the anterior walls of the foramen magnum. In life, they conduct the hypoglossal nerves.

RADIOLOGY OF THE SKULL

The student should be familiar with the five commonly used radiographic views of the skull. During such study a good quality skull should be available for reference. It should be emphasised that lateral and frontal views of the skull taken to show the *cranial* bones should not be used for detailed assessment of the *facial* bones or *sinuses*, even though these structures appear on the films. Specialised views and exposures are required for these examinations.

1. The lateral radiograph

For this view, the side of the head is placed against the X-ray film. When positioning the head, the interorbital line extending from the outer canthus of one eye to that of the other eye should be at right angles to the film. The bones forming the cranial vault should be inspected first, followed by an examination of the three cranial fossae (Figs. 1.7, 1.8, 1.9). Frontal, parietal, squamous temporal and occipital bones are visible on the lateral radiograph. The sutures are serrated and adjacent bone is often slightly more sclerotic than the rest of the vault in the adult. Both coronal and lambdoid sutures can usually be seen, and often the suture lines of both sides can be identified. When examining the lambdoid suture, its lower end will lead to the occipitomastoid suture (Fig. 1.9). This suture between the mastoid part of the temporal bone and the occipital bone must not be confused with a fracture of the posterior cranial fossa. The thickness of the calvaria of the adult skull varies from 3 to 8 mm, but is usually thicker than this over the occipital protuberance. The bones of the vault should be checked for vascular markings made by meningeal arteries, diploic veins, and certain venous sinuses. The groove for the anterior branch of the middle men-

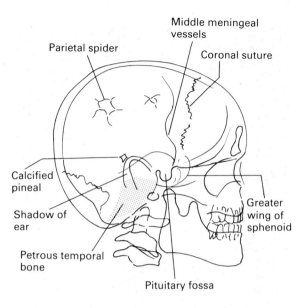

Fig. 1.7 Outline from a lateral radiograph of the skull

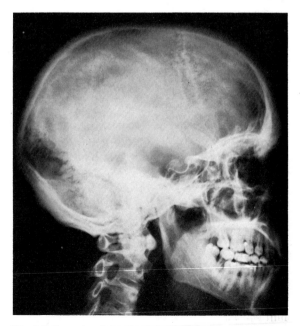

Fig. 1.8 Lateral radiograph of the skull

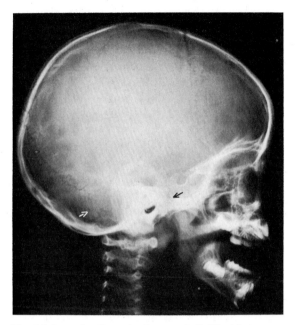

Fig. 1.9 Lateral radiograph of young skull. The black arrow points to the joint between the sphenoid and occipital bones. The white arrow points to the occipitomastoid suture.

ingeal artery often appears as a translucent line passing upwards behind the coronal suture. The groove for the posterior branch of the same artery may occasionally be found as it passes horizontally backwards to the shadow of the pinna. Frontal, parietal and occipital diploic veins are frequently seen on the lateral film. The parietal veins are usually particularly obvious, where they appear as stellate translucent shadows. Here, they are sometimes graphically described as the 'parietal spider'. Such patterns must not be confused with the picture of a depressed fracture. Arterial markings tend to narrow when traced peripherally from a bifurcation, whereas venous channel markings are often uneven in width. The superior sagittal sinus often gives rise to areas of translucency deep to the vault of the skull. The groove for the sigmoid sinus shows as a thick, curved line of translucency extending from the internal occipital protuberance forwards across the asterion and then down towards the acoustic meatus. Usually only the vascular markings of the side of the skull nearest the film are visible.

The outlines of the three cranial fossae forming the base of the cranial cavity are clearly visible on the lateral film. The air sinuses should be identified in the frontal bones, and their extent noted. Sometimes they are small, but when large may extend into the orbital plates of the frontal bone. Traced back across the anterior cranial fossa, the frontal bone is represented by the orbital plates, but right and left bones may not be accurately superimposed. Below the orbital plates a further opaque line represents the cribriform plate of the ethmoid. The floor of the anterior cranial fossa may be traced along the lesser wing of the sphenoid to the anterior clinoid process. The two anterior clinoids may be superimposed on one another in the film. The coronal suture and translucent line of the anterior branch of the middle meningeal artery sprout upwards from this part of the skull base.

A step over the anterior clinoid process leads to the middle cranial fossa. The most obvious part of this on the lateral film is the pituitary fossa. The anterior boundary of the fossa is the tuberculum sellae which appears as a prominent ridge in front of the fossa. In front of this ridge is a short sloping surface for the optic chiasma, the optic or chiasmatic groove. Behind, the pituitary fossa is limited by the dorsum sellae. Estimation of the size and shape of the pituitary fossa is required if a pituitary tumour is suspected. Below the pituitary fossa are the superimposed sphenoidal air sinuses. These vary considerably in size from individual to individual. At the front of these sinuses identify two white lines which curve upwards and cross the floor of the anterior cranial fossa. These are the greater wings of the sphenoid, and therefore represent the anterior boundaries of the middle cranial fossae. If these lines are traced backwards across the floor of the middle cranial fossa, a dense triangular area of bone is encountered, the petrous part of the temporal bone. The external acoustic meatus is sometimes visible as a translucency within this mass. Behind the meatus is the mastoid process, riddled with translucent air cells.

A step over the sharp ridge of the petrous temporal bone leads into the posterior cranial fossa. The anterior boundary of the fossa in the midline is the clivus, made up of both basisphenoid and basiocciput. A variable extent of the sloping clivus is visible on the lateral film, and can be found by tracing the line of the basisphenoid down from the posterior clinoid processes. Usually, however, much of the clivus is obscured by the petrous temporal bone. The cartilaginous joint between the basisphenoid and basiocciput is occasionally visible in subjects under the age of 25 years (Fig. 1.9). The foramen magnum cannot be identified on the lateral radiograph, but the position of its anterior boundary can be inferred by tracing the clivus downwards. Such a line hits the apex of the dens. Similarly, the position of the posterior boundary can also be estimated by tracing the occipital bone down to a point where its inner and outer tables merge.

CASE 4 (CONTINUED)

Among the initial investigations ordered for Dotty was a lateral radiograph of the skull. Examination of the pituitary region revealed that the fossa was enlarged, and the bone eroded (Fig. 1.10). It appeared as though there were two floors to the fossa, a radiological picture often called the 'double floor' sign. It indicates pituitary enlargement, one side enlarging more than the other. The initial radiological investigations therefore indicated that Dotty had a pituitary tumour. The extent and type of this tumour would need to be assessed, and the effect on vision investigated. (See Ch. 3 for continuation and conclusion.)

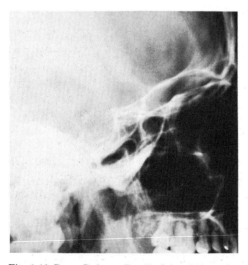

Fig. 1.10 Dotty Dobson. Detail of the pituitary fossa. (By kind permission of Dr B. M. Thomas, University College Hospital.)

2. Posteroanterior radiographs

On the lateral radiograph it was noted that the petrous temporal bone formed a dense shadow. On the frontal views the petrous parts of the temporal bones are also seen, but here they have an added disadvantage in that they obscure some important features of the skull bones. Radiographs taken with various degrees of head tilt are therefore used to examine all the bones of the skull. By tilting the skull, or the X-ray tube, the petrous shadows can be moved away from areas under examination. The petrous bones have been shaded in the diagrams of skull radiographs, and the student should pay particular attention to their positions in the various projections.

a. The straight posteroanterior radiograph

In this radiograph the beam is directed along the orbito-meatal line (Fig. 1.11A). This line runs from the external acoustic meatus to the outer canthus of the eye. In such a view the petrous ridges are projected into the orbits (Fig. 1.11B). The radiograph therefore cannot be used for information about the orbital bones or foramina. Both coronal and lambdoid sutures are visible in the vault, and are often almost superimposed one upon the other (Fig. 1.12). Thickness and symmetry of the bones of the vault should be compared on both sides. Usually the only vascular channel that is visible is a translucency produced by the superior sagittal sinus. The frontal air sinuses will be found on either side of the midline in the frontal region. They are often of unequal size and frequently the bony septum which separates the two sinuses is deviated towards one side or the other. The ethmoidal sinuses form a small translucent area between the medial wall of the orbit and the cavity of the nose.

b. Posteroanterior view with 15° tilt (Caldwell's projection)

With this degree of tilt, the shadows of the petrous temporal bones are carried down to be superimposed over the maxillary air sinuses rather than

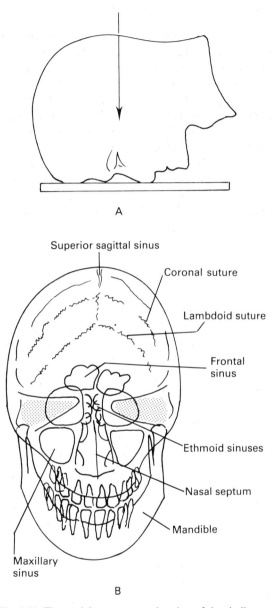

A

Superior sagittal sinus

Coronal suture

Lambdoid suture

Frontal sinus

Ethmoid sinuses

Nasal septum

Mandible

Maxillary sinus

B

Fig. 1.11 The straight posteroanterior view of the skull

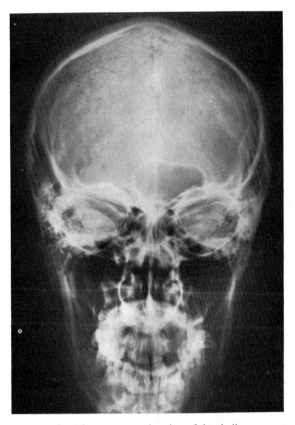

Fig. 1.12 Straight posteroanterior view of the skull

3. The anteroposterior view (Towne's projection)

In this projection the X-ray tube is tilted 30° caudally so that it looks towards the foramen magnum and occipital region. The view is used to look at the occipital region, dorsum sellae, and the petrous temporal bones (Figs. 1.15, 1.16). The most obvious feature on the film is the foramen magnum, the margins of which are easily defined. Within the foramen is the foreshortened shadow of the clivus and dorsum sellae. Above the foramen magnum the whole of the squamous occipital bone may be examined. It ends at the lambdoid suture on either side. The lower end of the lambdoid suture may be traced downwards to the suture between the occipital bone and the mastoid. As in the case of the lateral radiograph, this occipitomastoid suture must not be mistaken for a fracture. Beyond the lambdoid suture lie the parietal bones.

over the orbits (Figs. 1.13). In the orbit, the superior orbital fissure will be seen between the greater and lesser wings of the sphenoid (Fig. 1.14). The optic canal is sometimes visible on its medial side.

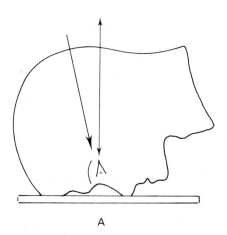

A

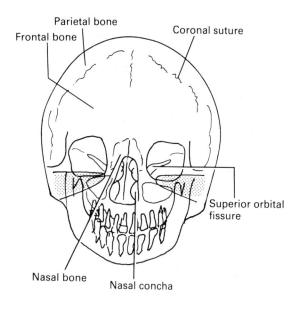

B

Fig. 1.13 Posteroanterior with 15° tilt (Caldwell's projection)

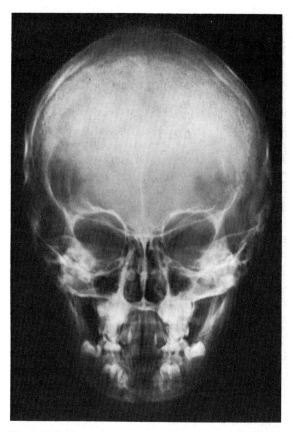

Fig. 1.14 Radiograph of the skull — Caldwell's projection

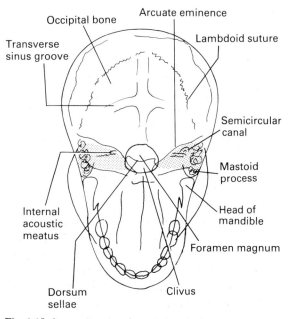

Fig. 1.15 Anteroposterior view (Towne's projection)

The occipital protuberance is seen as a midline opacity above the foramen magnum. Dense lines radiate laterally from the protuberance on either side, and in the midline above. The horizontal shadows represent the edges of the body sulci which contain the transverse sinuses. On either side of the foramen magnum the dense shadows of the petrous temporal bones will be seen. The petrous ridge or superior border of this bone should be carefully examined, because the arcuate

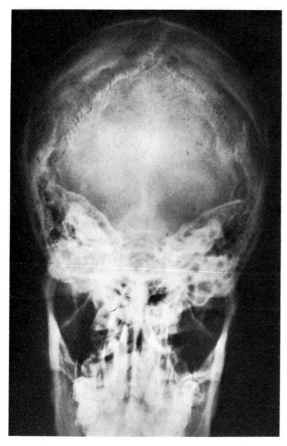

Fig. 1.16 Radiograph of the skull — Towne's projection

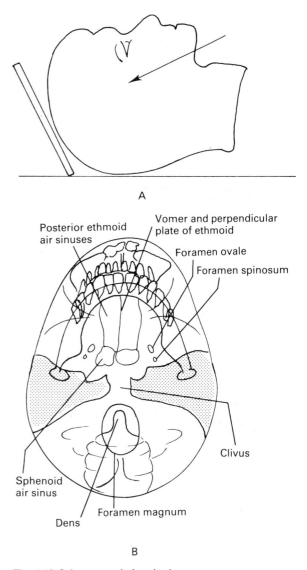

Fig. 1.17 Submentovertical projection

eminence is sometimes visible on it, with a small lucent area formed by the anterior semicircular canal below. It is also occasionally possible to identify a small translucent shadow below the canal made by the cochlea. The internal acoustic meatus may also be found entering the bone medial to the arcuate eminence.

4. Submentovertical view

This type of radiograph is used when details of the base of the cranial cavity are required (Fig. 1.17). It may also be used to demonstrate some features of the mandible and the zygomatic arches (see Ch. 12). For now, identify only the structures in the base of the cranial cavity. As in the previous view, the foramen magnum is the obvious place to

start (Fig. 1.18). Within it is the shadow of the dens, and on either side the condyles are visible. In front of the foramen magnum is the clivus. The cartilaginous joint between basisphenoid and basiocciput is clearly seen on this view in subjects under the age of 25 years. Identify on either side the triangular densities of the petrous temporal bones. In front of the apex of the bone is the foramen lacerum. Turn your attention to the groove between the petrous temporal bone behind, and the greater wing of sphenoid in front. The lucent

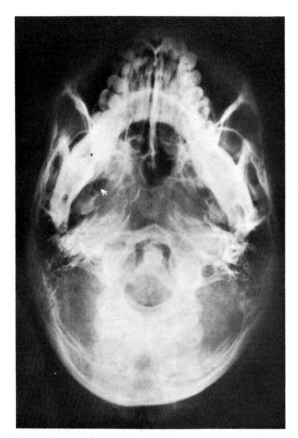

Fig. 1.18 Radiograph of the skull — submentovertical projection. The white arrow indicates the foramen ovale.

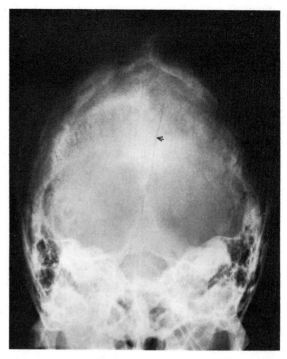

Fig. 1.19 Tom Talbott. Radiograph — Towne's projection. Black arrow — fracture.

auditory tube can be identified along the junction of these two bones. Several foramina may be seen in the submentovertical projection. In the greater wing of the sphenoid look for the foramen ovale (Fig. 1.18), and the foramen spinosum behind it. In the petrous temporal bone the lucent area formed by the carotid canal may be found. The jugular foramen is usually not seen in this projection, but it can be brought into view by further tilting of the X-ray tube.

CASES 1, 2 AND 3 (CONTINUED)

The anteroposterior radiograph of Tom's skull showed a fracture of the occipital bone (Fig. 1.19). There was no skull fracture on Dick's radiographs. Harry's posteroanterior radiograph showed two oblique fractures of the right frontal bone. These fractures extended to the orbital margin (Fig. 1.20).

It was obvious that Tom would need urgent surgical treatment, which was impossible in the small

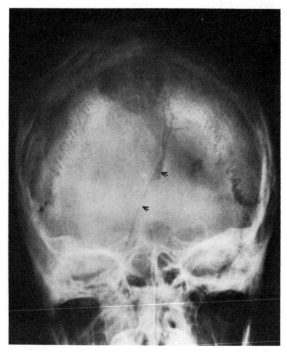

Fig. 1.20 Harry Harper. Radiograph — straight posteroanterior view. Black arrows — fracture.

medical centre. All three patients, accompanied by
the attending physician, would need to be trans-
ported to the nearest hospital centre. Evacuation
by helicopter was arranged, and they arrived at the
hospital 90 minutes later.

THE NEONATAL SKULL

The bones which form the case around the developing brain ossify in one of two ways. The flat
bones of the vault develop by membranous
ossification. The bones which form the cranial
base, however, ossify from a number of cartilaginous plates (Fig. 1.21). The middle part of the
skull base from the foramen magnum to the
ethmoid is formed from several plates. On either
side of this, lateral cartilages give rise to the lesser
and greater wings of the sphenoid, and the petro-
mastoid part of the temporal bones.

The physician may be called upon to examine
the skull of a neonate or young child, therefore
differences between the adult and neonatal skull
should be carefully noted. At birth, the skull is
large when it is compared to other parts of the
skeleton. Closer examination will reveal that it is
the cranial part of the skull which is large, and that
the facial part is relatively small. The maxillae,
which form a major part of the facial skeleton, are
small. Although there are tooth germs present in
the maxillae, the maxillary air sinuses are no more
than small slits beneath the floor of the orbits.
These features, together with the small size of the
mandible and non-erupted teeth, account for the
size and proportions of the neonatal face. Check
these features on Figure 1.9. Although this radiograph is of a child older than a neonate, it still
shows many of the features of the young skull.
The bones of the vault have no diploë at this stage
in development: this appears during the fourth
year of life. Although the size of the calvaria is
large, it is still not completely ossified. The frontal
bone is in two halves separated by a midline metopic suture. Segments of the fibrous membrane
which formed the primitive vault still remain in
the angles between the flat bones. These areas are
called 'fontanelles' (Fig. 1.22). The anterior fontanelle is the largest and is found at the junction
of the metopic, sagittal and coronal sutures. A
smaller posterior fontanelle is located at the junc-

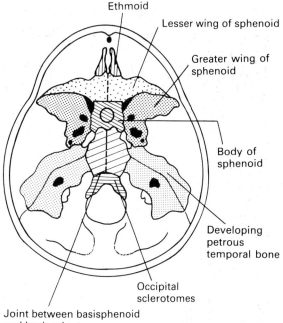

Fig. 1.21 Development of the skull base

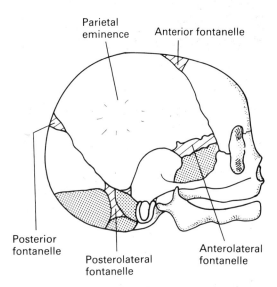

Fig. 1.22 The neonatal skull

tion of the lambdoid and sagittal sutures. The anterolateral or sphenoidal fontanelle is found at the
junction of the parietal, frontal, sphenoid and
squamous temporal bones, and is the site of the
future pterion. A posterolateral or mastoid fonta-

nelle is wedged between the parietal, occipital and mastoid temporal bones. Growth of the bones of the vault of the skull is rapid during the first year of life, and continues at a slower rate until about the seventh year of life. By this time the vault of the skull has reached almost adult dimensions. This growth of the vault reflects a similar increase in the size of the enclosed brain. At birth the brain is growing at a rapid rate, most of the neurones being present. A further addition of glial cells occurs during the first few months after birth. The brain is 80% of its adult size at the age of 2 years. Indeed, one of the best assessments of brain size in the young child is head circumference. This measurement is taken as the widest occipitofrontal circumference. Serial measurements may be plotted with reference to normal head-size charts. A massive rate of growth may indicate increased intracranial pressure, and a slow rate may signal a problem with brain development. Such observations, however, must always take into account genetic factors involved in determining head size. It is therefore important to note the size and shape of the heads of both parents. Most of the growth in the vault takes place by ossification at the adjacent margins of the bones, i.e. at the sutures. In the process of rapid growth in the first and second years of life this results in the closure of the fontanelles. The anterolateral and posterior fontanelles close during the first 3 months of life. The posterolateral is closed by the end of the first year. The anterior fontanelle, because of its large size, closes later at about 18 months. Occasionally, separate centres of ossification occur in the membrane of the fontanelles, and produce sutural bones. This is not uncommon in the region of the posterior fontanelle. Such bones in the anterolateral fontanelle are called 'epipteric bones'. By the time all the fontanelles are closed, late in the second year, the sutures are interlocked, and expansion of the vault during subsequent years is produced by bone absorption on the deep surface of the bones and accretion on the superficial surface. During this process, inner and outer tables of the flat bones are formed with intervening diploë.

Most of the bony elements making up both temporal and occipital bones are separate in the neonatal skull. (Details of the development of the temporal bone are given in Ch. 4.) The occipital bone of the newborn consists of four parts (Fig. 1.23). The flat squamous section of the bone ossifies in membrane above the highest nuchal line and in cartilage below it, but union of these two parts is not always complete by birth. Two lateral sections of the occipital bone ossify in cartilage at the sides of the foramen magnum, each bearing a large section of the occipital condyle. The basilar part of the occipital bone, in front of the foramen magnum, also ossifies in cartilage. The occipital bone is fully united by the age of 6 years. Growth in length of the base of the skull takes place mainly at the synchondrosis between the basiocciput and the basisphenoid (see Figs. 1.9, 1.21). This fuses sometime between the ages of 15 and 25 years. Some growth in length also takes place in the synchondrosis between the ethmoid and sphenoid bones.

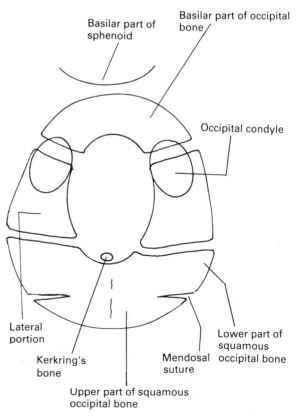

Fig. 1.23 Development of the occipital bone

During birth, both the sutures and the anterior and posterior fontanelles may be palpated on vaginal examination. Several measurements of the fetal skull are useful in obstetrics (Fig. 1.24). The biparietal diameter is the distance between the two parietal tuberosities and is the largest transverse diameter of the skull. Its average measurement is 9.5 cm. The bitemporal diameter, between the two temporal bones, is the shortest diameter and is usually of the order of 8 cm. The presenting part of the fetal head depends on the degree of flexion of the neck. Normally, with the head fully flexed, it is the suboccipitobregmatic diameter which presents. This diameter is only 9.5 cm long, with a suboccipitobregmatic circumference of about 32–34 cm. The bisacromial diameter between the shoulders is 33–34 cm. Thus, if the head gets through the birth canal in this position,

and occipital bones passing under the parietal bone edges. Compression in one direction is accompanied by expansion in another, so that the volume of the skull is not reduced and the underlying brain is not damaged. As the fetal head descends, pressure of the maternal cervical ring causes obstruction to venous return in the fetal scalp. This part of the scalp becomes oedematous, and a swelling called a 'caput succedaneum' results (Fig. 1.25A, B). The caput forms during labour after the membranes have ruptured, and its location depends on the presenting part of the head. In the common left occipitoanterior position, the caput forms on the vertex and to the right of the sagittal suture. The caput, present at birth, disappears rapidly over the subsequent 24–36 hours. The caput must be distinguished from a cephalhaematoma (Fig. 1.25C). This is a traumatic

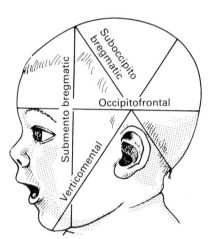

Fig. 1.24 Diameters of the neonatal skull

the shoulders should present no difficulty. With the head fully extended there will be a face presentation, with a submentobregmatic diameter of 9.5 cm. Positions between full flexion and full extension will present larger diameters, such as the occipitofrontal and the verticomental distances. The latter diameter is the largest of the anteroposterior diameters, and is the diameter found in a brow presentation.

During labour the fetal head changes its shape in order to adapt to the unyielding maternal pelvis. Overlapping of the bones takes place, the frontal

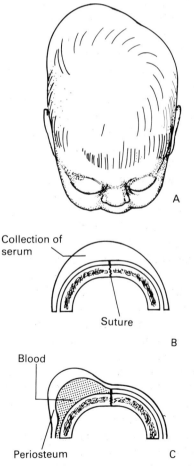

Fig. 1.25 A: Caput succedaneum. B: Caput in section. C: Cephalhaematoma.

haemorrhage under the periosteum of one or more bones of the skull, usually the parietal bone. The haemorrhage does not cross suture lines because it is deep to the periosteum, and in this way may be distinguished from a caput. Absorption of the haematoma is slow and may take as long as 12 weeks.

RADIOLOGICAL ANATOMY OF THE SKULL AT BIRTH

In the neonate and young child, the bones which form the cranial vault are thin, for they have not yet formed separate inner and outer tables. The junctions between bones of the newborn skull should be carefully traced, together with the regions of the fontanelles. In the base of the skull note should be made of several primary cartilaginous joints (synchondroses).

On the posteroanterior projection of the newborn skull the anterior fontanelle appears as a large diamond-shaped defect. From the lower point of the fontanelle the metopic suture can be traced towards the nose. Figure 1.26 shows the radiograph of an 18-month-old child. The metopic suture is still visible. The suture closes sometime during the first few years of life, but may occasionally remain into adult life.

On the lateral radiograph, the coronal sutures appear wide in the neonatal skull, and end above in the anterior fontanelle. At the lower end of the coronal suture is the anterolateral fontanelle. The lambdoid suture extends obliquely downwards and forwards from the posterior fontanelle to the posterolateral (mastoid) fontanelle. From the lower end of the lambdoid suture a small slit extends backwards; this so-called 'Mendosal suture' is all that remains of the joint between the upper and lower parts of the squamous occipital bone. This is visible in the radiograph in Figure 1.27 of a child of 18 months. Note also in this radiograph that there are no separate tables, and that the bones of the vault are thin. The frontal and maxillary air sinuses are rudimentary in the skull, and the mastoid process has not developed.

The occipital bone may be examined on the verticosubmental and Towne's views. In front of the foramen magnum the basal part of the occipital

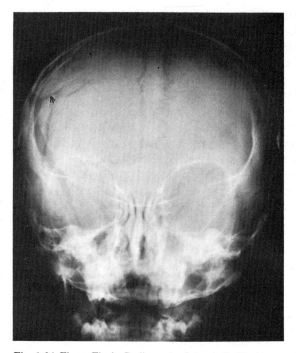

Fig. 1.26 Flossy Flook. Radiograph of the skull. Black arrow — fracture.

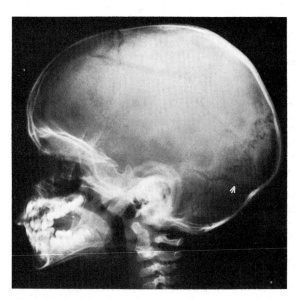

Fig. 1.27 Flossy Flook. Lateral radiograph of the skull. The white arrow points to the Mendosal suture.

bone is attached to the basal part of the sphenoid bone by means of the spheno-occipital synchondrosis. These bones overlap in the Towne's view, but the synchondrosis is visible in the submentovertical projection, and in the lateral view of the skull (see Fig. 1.9). All the synchondroses between the various parts of the occipital bone unite by the time the child is 6 years of age, and by the age of 25 years the synchondrosis between the basiocciput and basisphenoid is usually united. Sutures begin to fuse during the third decade of life, but there is a great variation in the extent to which this takes place.

CASE 5

Fanny Flook was a 23-year-old mother. She had been separated from her husband for two years, and had been trying to bring up two toddlers and an 18-month-old child, Flossy, in a small one-bedroom apartment. She brought little Flossy to the accident unit with a story that the child had accidentally fallen out of her cot onto the head. On examination, Flossy had severe bruising and swelling over the right temple. A careful examination, however, revealed that she also had bruising of the right wrist, chest, and circular burn marks on the buttocks. After initial examination she was sent for skull, wrist and chest radiographs.

The radiograph of the skull showed extensive fractures through the right temporal and parietal bones with some overlap of the fragments (Figs. 1.26–1.28), Wrist and chest radiographs were normal.

Flossy was admitted to hospital after the examination had been completed. After further conversation, the mother was referred to the social worker on duty. The picture of multiple injuries and burn marks indicated that poor Flossy might have been a 'battered baby'. Maltreatment of young children by relatives is not uncommon, and the student must be on the lookout for such cases. With gentle questioning, Fanny admitted that she was unable to cope with the children, and had struck Flossy several times after the child had a long bout of crying. The marks on the buttocks were from cigarette burns, inflicted a few days before examination. Flossy made a good recovery, in spite of the severe trauma.

Fanny needed help for many years, but her health deteriorated, and she was unable to continue to look after her children. Eventually a new home had to be found for Flossy.

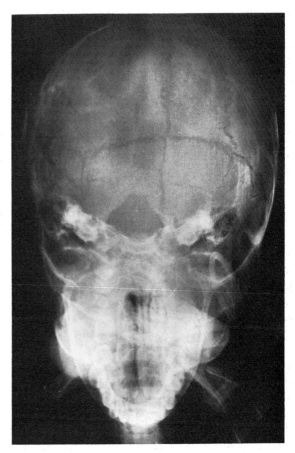

Fig. 1.28 Flossy Flook. Radiograph of the occipital region.

COMPUTER TOMOGRAPHY

Geoffrey Hounsfield revolutionised the investigation of cranial disease with the introduction of computed tomography (CT) in the early 1970s. Hounsfield's original description in 1973 in the *British Journal of Radiology* (46: 1016–1022) gives an excellent description of the working of the instrument. What is shown on the picture is *not* a direct radiograph but a mathematical reconstruction of it. The X-ray tube passes back and forth recording a series of tomographic slices through the head in either the horizontal or coronal plane (Fig. 1.29). Other planes are used for examining special areas such as the pituitary fossa and the petrous temporal bone. The computer makes a reconstruction from many measurements of absorp-

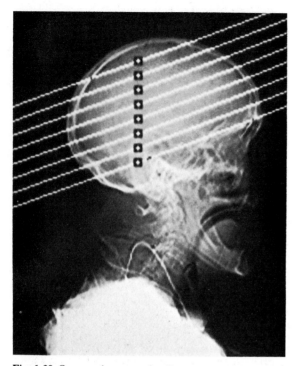

Fig. 1.29 Computed tomography slices

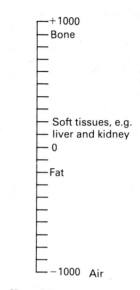

Fig. 1.30 The Hounsfield scale

tion densities and the position and angle of the beam. Cuts are usually made several millimetres apart. Numerous degrees of 'greyness', many not discernable to the human eye, are available on the tomogram. They are measured on the Hounsfield scale of CT numbers (Fig. 1.30). On this arbitrary scale, air is designated −1000 Hounsfield units (HU), and appears black. Water is 0 HU, and bone about +1000 HU. The computer can create a detailed image at any part of the scale to selectively look at air, soft tissues or bone. This selection is known as creating a 'window'. During examination of the chest, for example, the window could be set around a low negative value if the air-filled lungs are to be examined. On the other hand, a positive value would be used if the soft tissues of the lungs or thorax needed examination.

Contrast enhancement increases the amount of information which can be obtained from many scans. The technique involves the intravenous injection of an iodine-based compound. Slices are made before and after the injection. At other times metrizamide is introduced into the cerebrospinal fluid by either lumbar or suboccipital puncture. This enhances the appearance of the chiasmatic cistern above the pituitary fossa and of the cerebellopontine angle during investigations of the petrous temporal bone. The convention for looking at a CT scan is illustrated in Figure 1.31. The horizontal slice is looked at from *below*. Right and left sides are therefore as marked on the diagram. As you follow the case histories through the next few chapters you will be introduced to computed tomograms. Other imaging techniques, apart from

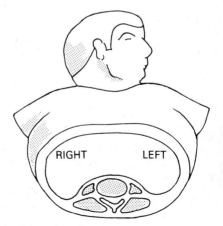

Fig. 1.31 Orientation of a CT slice

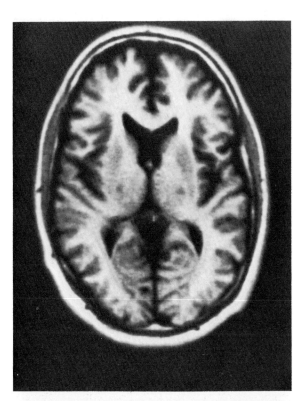

Fig. 1.32 MRI scan. Transverse inversion recovery image of a normal adult brain. (By kind permission of Dr Jackie Pennock and the NMR Unit of the Royal Postgraduate Medical School, Hammersmith Hospital.)

Fig. 1.33   A: MRI scan. Inversion recovery image showing a tumour in the thalamus (dark area). B: MRI scan. A tumour is highlighted (bright area) after injection of contrast agent (Gadolinium DTPA—Schering AG, Berlin). (By kind permission of Dr Jackie Pennock and the NMR Unit of The Royal Postgraduate Medical School, Hammersmith Hospital.)

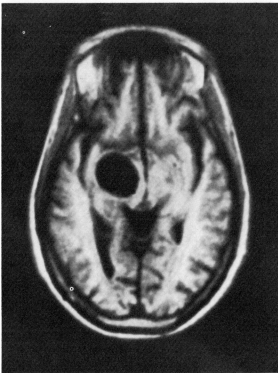

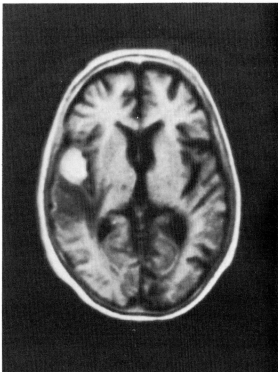

A   B

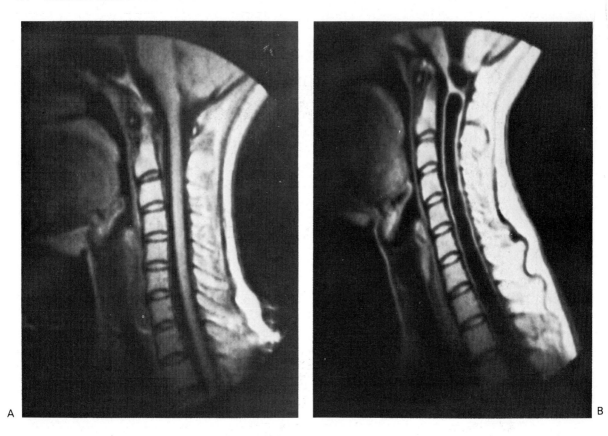

A   B

Fig. 1.34 A: MRI scan. Sagittal image showing a normal cervical spine. B: MRI scan. Sagittal image of the cervical cord of a patient with hydromyelia. (Note the dark central part of the spinal cord.)

computer tomography, are available. These include ultrasound (US), nuclear imaging, and magnetic resonance imaging (MRI). The student will be introduced to ultrasound scans and nuclear imaging in Volume 3. Magnetic resonance imaging is a non-invasive, non-ionising technique. Images are produced when the patient is placed in a magnetic field and a radio frequency wave is pulsed through the tissues. This manipulates the nuclei of the hydrogen ions, or protons, in the tissues of the body. Protons normally spin around a fixed axis like a child's spinning top. You will recall, however, that as well as spinning, a top also precesses around the axis of the spin, the whole top moving in this motion. If protons are placed in a magnetic field, they line up parallel to the field and precess around it just like the top precesses around the vertical gravitational field. The rate. of frequency of precession is proportional to the

magnetic field. In magnetic resonance imaging, a radio frequency of the same frequency as the proton precession is beamed onto the patient and this alters the proton alignment. At this frequency they absorb energy from the beam, resonance absorption, and align themselves relative to the magnetic field. If a stronger radio pulse is applied at the same time as the magnetic field, it is even possible to flip them over 180°. When the irradiating frequency is switched off, the nuclei have surplus energy which they radiate to their surroundings at the same resonant frequency. One by one the nuclei fall back to their original alignment or 'relax', and the tissue re-emits its resonant frequency. It is this that is measured. The length of time for relaxation depends on the environment of the protons, some substances producing a faster decay time than others. It is thus possible to identify chemicals in the tissue. When the patient is placed in the machine, a magnetic field gradient is applied. This enables the position of anatomical structures to be identified from the frequency of the emitted signal. The proton concentration (amount of water) in the tissue can also be measured from the size of the signal, and the relaxation time from the decay of the signal. With this information a picture is generated of either proton concentration distribution or relaxation time distribution in the tissues. Composite pictures may also be produced. Figures 1.32, 1.33, and 1.34 are MRI scans. You will notice that although much of the information they give is similar to that obtained by computed tomography, they give detailed information of the soft tissues such as the brain. Figure 1.32 is a transverse section of a head, and the structure of the cerebral hemispheres, including the grey and white matter, can be seen. Figure 1.33A is also a horizontal section, but there is a large black hole (a tumour) in the thalamus. The use of contrast agents during computed tomography was noted. They are also used during magnetic resonance imaging. Figure 1.33B shows a tumour highlighted by injection of contrast medium. Figure 1.34A shows a sagittal image of the cervical spine and posterior cranial fossa. Compare this with Figure 1.34B which is a scan from a patient who has an increased amount of fluid in the central canal of the spinal cord (hydromyelia).

The student often finds the study of the skull laborious. Indeed, there is no simple way of learning about it. If, however, the student is prepared to spend some time studying skull radiographs with the help of a good quality skull, the rewards will be great in later years when he is confronted with cases of head injury and cranial disease.

2

THE CRANIAL CAVITY

THE MENINGES

The brain and spinal cord are surrounded by three meningeal layers. The outermost fibrous membrane, the dura mater, is separated from the middle layer, the arachnoid, by the subdural space. The innermost membrane, the pia mater, is intimately associated with the surface of both brain and spinal cord. Between the arachnoid and pia is a subarachnoid space containing cerebrospinal fluid.

1. The dura

The cerebral dura lines the inside of the skull and is continuous through the foramen magnum with the spinal dura. Unlike its spinal counterpart, however, much of the cranial dura is fused with the periosteum of the cranial bones. Indeed, at the skull base and over the suture lines the dura and periosteum cannot be separated. Even microscopically there is no line of division between these two membranes. Thus, at places where this fusion is strong, removal of the dura strips down to bare bone. Four folds of dura extend into the cranial cavity between the parts of the brain, and support the brain. The falx cerebri is a sickle-shaped fold in the mid-sagittal plane (Fig. 2.1). It is attached in front to the crista galli, foramen caecum and frontal crest. Its upper convex margin is attached to the cranial vault as far back as the internal occipital protruberance. The lower concave margin of the falx presents a sharp edge, but posteriorly it is attached to the tentorium cerebelli. The tentorium cerebelli, like the falx, also has attached

and free margins. As its name implies, it is a tented structure with its highest line at the attachment to the falx. The outer margin is attached on each side to the lips of the transverse sulcus. This attachment may be traced forwards along the superior edge of the petrous temporal bone as far as the posterior clinoid process. The free border of the tentorium encloses a large opening called the 'tentorial incisure', through which the middle and posterior cranial fossae are continuous. This sharp edge of tentorium, as it is traced forwards, *crosses* the attached margin to reach the *anterior* clinoid process. The sella turcica is roofed by a fold of dura called the 'diaphragma sellae'. This is attached in front to the tuberculum sellae and behind to the dorsum sellae. Centrally it has a small opening through which the pituitary stalk passes. A small fold of dura, the falx cerebelli, is found in the midline of the posterior cranial fossa below the tentorium cerebelli.

The dura covering the floor of the cranial fossae has a rich sensory nerve supply, while that covering the vault is less sensitive. These sensory nerves also contain sympathetic vasoconstrictor fibres. Anterior cranial fossa dura receives most of its supply from ethmoidal nerves. The middle cranial fossa dura receives meningeal branches from the maxillary and mandibular divisions of the trigeminal nerve. Branches of the ophthalmic division of the trigeminal nerve sweep backwards across the middle cranial fossa floor to the tentorium cerebelli. This group of nerves, referred to as the 'recurrent tentorial nerve', supplies dura of the middle cranial fossa and the tentorium cerebelli. The posterior cranial fossa dura is innervated

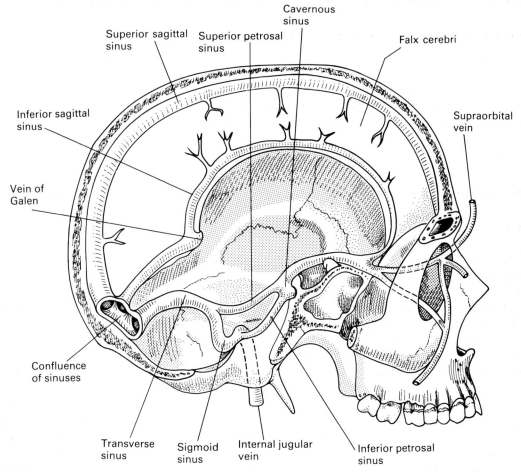

Fig. 2.1 The venous sinuses

by meningeal branches of the upper cervical nerves. These enter the fossa through the foramen magnum, jugular foramen, and the hypoglossal canal. Some of these nerves hitch-hike for a short distance along cranial nerves such as the vagus and hypoglossal nerves. The fibrous dura requires little blood supply, and the vessels called 'meningeal' are mostly destined to be nutrient arteries to the vault of the skull. The relationship of the arteries to the dura is important. Being nutrient arteries to the bone, they lie outside the dura, and are therefore described as being extradural in position.

CASES 1, 2 AND 3 (CONTINUED FROM CHAPTER 1)

Tom, Dick and Harry, the subjects of the first three case studies of Chapter 1, were evacuated from the desert oil rig after the accident.

Tom
Although Tom's condition was grave, he tolerated the journey well. Arrangements were made for blood transfusion. Examination by the neurosurgeon included a CT scan of the head (Fig. 2.2). A large extracerebral collection of blood was seen on the right side, pushing the brain and its ventricles to the left. Small intracerebral haemorrhages were seen on the opposite side of the brain. This type of damage, occurring on the side opposite to the main lesion, is called a 'contre coup' injury. With the blood transfusion in progress, Tom was prepared for surgery by the anaesthetist.

Operation notes
The general surgeon opened the left upper abdomen and found a small amount of blood in the

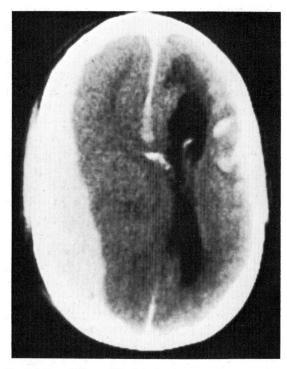

Fig. 2.2 Tom Talbott. CT of the head.

peritoneal cavity. The spleen had been ruptured, but the haemorrhage had been contained within its capsule. The splenic hilus was clamped and a splenectomy performed. The abdominal wound was quickly closed.

The neurosurgeon proceeded with a right craniotomy. A vertical incision was made half-way between the orbit and the external acoustic meatus. The incision was taken through skin and temporalis muscle. Exposure of the bone in this region revealed a small crack, not detected by radiography. A burr hole was made adjacent to the small fracture, the rotating burr piercing outer and inner tables of bone. Bone dust and chips were washed away with saline during the procedure. As soon as the bone had been removed, a tarry clot was visible outside the dura (Fig. 2.3). More bone was nibbled away to give a wider exposure, and the clot traced down towards the floor of the middle cranial fossa. A small extradural branch of the middle meningeal artery was bleeding, and this was stopped by diathermy coagulation. (In severe bleeds, it is occasionally necessary to plug the foramen spinosum, and occlude the main trunk of the middle meningeal artery.) The oozing points of the bone edges were stopped with Horsley's bone wax by squeezing it into the diploic spaces. The extradural clot was gently evacuated.

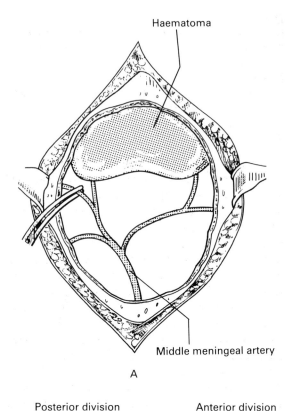

A

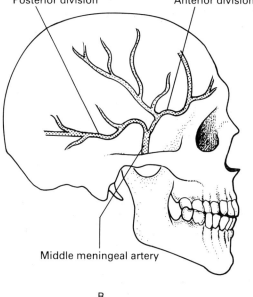

B

Fig. 2.3 A: Tom Talbott. Operation for an extradural haematoma. B: Surface marking of the middle meningeal artery.

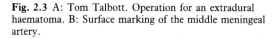

The temporalis muscle, galea and scalp were closed with sutures.

Dick

Dick's condition had remained stable since evacuation, and he was admitted for observation.

Harry

Harry was also in fairly good shape, but was also admitted for observation.

2. The arachnoid and subarachnoid space

The arachnoid is separated from the dura by a subdural space, and from the pia by the subarachnoid space. This latter space contains cerebrospinal fluid (CSF). Many of the blood vessels which supply the brain have to cross the space. In certain regions around the base of the brain, the arachnoid is widely separated from the pia, and here the CSF pools in the form of cisterns (Fig. 2.4). These large lakes of CSF are continuous with each other and the general cerebrospinal fluid. The cisterna magna or cerebellomedullary cistern is a pool located in the angle between the medulla and overhanging cerebellum. In front of the pons is a large lake of CSF called the 'pontine cistern'. This lies deep to the arachnoid covering the clivus, and is traversed by the basilar artery. The lateral recesses of the pontine cistern, or cerebellopontine cisterns, may be distorted by posterior fossa lesions. The pontine cistern is continuous below with a med-

ullary cistern which lies in front of the medulla. Traced upwards, the pontine cistern leads into another pool called the 'interpeduncular cistern', and this contains the circulus arteriosus of Willis. The interpeduncular cistern extends forwards to the optic chiasma, and a pool of CSF associated with this structure forms the pre- and post-chiasmatic cisterns. Although difficult to determine, it is probable that the arachnoid and CSF do not extend through the diaphragma sellae around the pituitary. Above the chiasmatic cisterns, stretching between the two cerebral hemispheres, is a pool of CSF related to the corpus callosum, and the anterior cerebral arteries traverse the CSF in this region. Further laterally, the arachnoid bridges the lateral sulcus to form the cistern of the lateral fossa, and the middle cerebral artery is found here. Traced back over the corpus callosum the subarachnoid space leads to the interval between the splenium of the corpus and the upper surface of the cerebellum. The cistern of the great cerebral vein lies here, and houses the vein of the same name. Extensions of this cistern around the sides of the colliculi form the cisterna ambiens on each side.

One of the first methods used for investigating the cisterns was air encephalography. During this procedure, 10 ml of air is injected into the CSF by

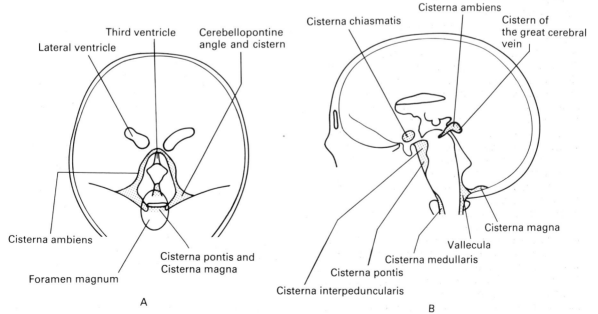

A

B

Fig. 2.4 The cisterns. A: Anteroposterior view. B: Lateral view.

means of a lumbar puncture. It tracks up to the fourth ventricle and can be identified by a lateral radiograph of the skull. More air is then injected and some CSF withdrawn. If the head is then extended the subarachnoid cisterns will fill with air. Finally, it is possible to fill the ventricular system of the brain with air. This type of investigation is still used in conjunction with computed tomography (see Fig. 4.20). The cisterns can also be outlined by positive contrast introduced into the CSF.

CSF is produced by the choroid plexuses within the ventricles of the brain. It escapes into the subarachnoid space through three foramina in the fourth ventricle. In the midline is the median aperture of Magendie through which CSF reaches the cisterna magna. On either side are lateral apertures of Luschka, and CSF flows through these to the pontine cistern. Although some CSF may drain back into the venous system through vertebral venous plexuses, most returns by means of specialised structures called 'arachnoid granulations' (Fig. 2.5). These are mainly found in association with the superior sagittal sinus, and with venous lacunae on the sides of the sinus. A few are found in other major sinuses. Close inspection of

an arachnoid granulation shows it to be composed of a small projection of arachnoid, the arachnoid villus, through the dura into the venous sinus. The surface of the arachnoid villus is covered with an endothelial lining continuous with that of the venous sinus itself. Fluid passes from the CSF to the venous system by filtration, although minute valvular openings in the villi have also been postulated.

CASES 1, 2 AND 3 (CONTINUED)

Tom
Tom was returned to intensive care for observation.

Dick
Dick passed an uneventful first night, and developed no problems.

Harry
Harry, however, complained of a little watery discharge from the nose during the night. Examination showed a small amount of fluid draining from the right nostril. The fluid contained glucose, and was therefore assumed to be CSF. Head injuries sometimes result in tears of the basal dura

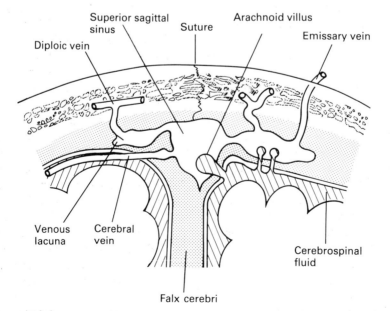

Fig. 2.5 The superior sagittal sinus

and arachnoid. Harry had fractures of the frontal bone, and these probably extended into the anterior cranial fossa. Fracture of the cribriform plate of the ethmoid allowed CSF to drain into the nose. This condition is called 'rhinorrhoea'. Harry was given large doses of antibiotics, because of the danger of infection spreading from the nose to the meninges. The discharge dried up within 3 days, and Harry had no further problems. If the dural tear is severe, air sometimes replaces some of the CSF around the cerebral hemispheres, and can be seen on a radiograph. This condition is called an 'aerocele'. Dural tears may also occur with fractures of the petrous temporal bone. This leads to discharge of CSF from the ear, a condition called 'otorrhoea'.

3. The pia

The cerebral pia is intimately associated with the surface of the brain, covering the gyri and dipping into the sulci. In certain situations, the walls of the ventricles are composed of epithelium (ependyma) only. Here, pia is invaginated into the ventricles as the tela choroidea. With the ependyma, this forms the choroid plexuses of the ventricles. The choroid plexuses are responsible for the formation of CSF.

THE VENOUS SINUSES

A system of venous sinuses is closely associated with the cranial dura. Some sinuses are located between the dura and periosteum, while others are enclosed between the folds of dura. The sinuses drain blood from the brain and from the bones of the skull (see Fig. 2.1). They also have connections at certain points with veins on the outside of the skull. The sinuses contain no valves and have no muscular tissue in their walls. They are lined with endothelium which is continuous with that of the veins into which they drain. The sinuses eventually drain into the internal jugular vein through the jugular foramen, and into the vertebral venous plexuses through the foramen magnum.

The superior sagittal sinus starts at the front of the falx cerebri near the crista galli. As it runs backwards in the sagittal plane it grooves the inner table of the frontal, parietal and occipital bones. At the internal occipital protuberance it usually deviates to the right to become continuous with

the right transverse sinus. This is not always the case, however, for occasionally the sinus joins the left transverse sinus. The dilated posterior end of the superior sagittal sinus, as it joins the right transverse sinus, receives blood from an occipital sinus and is also connected to the left transverse sinus. This confluence of sinuses is known as the 'torcular Herophili'. ('Torcular' is derived from the Latin word for a winepress. Herophilus was a Greek physician and anatomist who lived in Alexandria around 300 BC, and is often described as 'the father of anatomy', for he performed dissections and made many anatomical descriptions.) Venous lacunae are located on either side of the superior sagittal sinus, and diploic and meningeal veins open into them, together with the occasional emissary vein (Fig. 2.5). The superior sagittal sinus also receives blood from the external cerebral veins, the superior set of which enter the sinus obliquely against the current of blood.

The inferior sagittal sinus is found in the free edge of the falx cerebri. It starts about a third of the way along the falx as a small venous channel, and continues as far as the junction between the falx and tentorium. Here, it continues as the straight sinus. This passes to the confluence of sinuses, where it usually drains into the left transverse sinus. There is a communication between this junction and the right transverse sinus. At its anterior end, the straight sinus receives the great cerebral vein of Galen. This drains the deep parts of the cerebral hemispheres together with some drainage from the cerebellum and brain stem. Superior cerebellar veins also drain into the straight sinus. The typical formation of the transverse sinuses has already been described, but many variations occur. Each transverse sinus is large, and begins at the internal occipital protuberance (Fig. 2.6). In its course laterally it deeply grooves the occipital bone, and reaches the petrous part of the temporal bone. Each sinus lies in the attached edge of the tentorium cerebelli. The transverse sinuses receive inferior cerebral and cerebellar veins. Each transverse sinus also receives the superior petrosal sinus and then curves downwards towards the jugular foramen as the sigmoid sinus. The sigmoid sinus grooves the mastoid part of the temporal bone, and is separated from the mastoid air cells by a thin plate of bone. A mastoid emissary

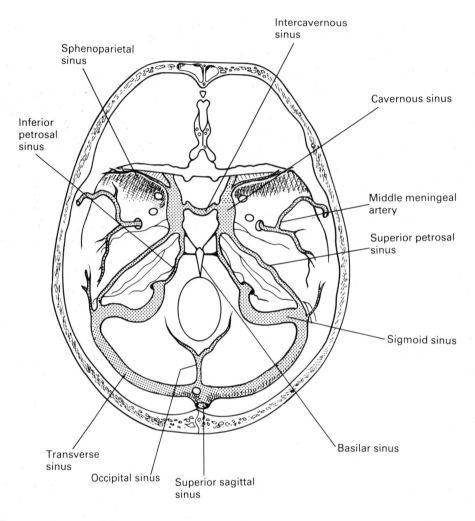

Fig. 2.6 The venous sinuses

vein often acts as a communication between the sigmoid sinus and veins on the outside of the skull.

The student should pay particular attention to the cavernous sinuses, for they are placed on each side of the sphenoid bone in close relationship to vital structures such as the pituitary, the internal carotid artery and certain cranial nerves. Numerous trabeculae traverse the cavity of each sinus to give it a spongy form. Each sinus starts in front at the superior orbital fissure. It will be recalled that the free margin of the tentorium passes as far as the anterior clinoid process. Dura between this ridge and the diaphragma sellae constitutes the roof of the cavernous sinus. The posterior boundary of the roof is formed by the attached edge of the tentorium which extends to the posterior clinoid process. Flow into the front of the cavernous sinus comes from the ophthalmic veins. Such an input constitutes a communication between the venous system on the outside of the skull and the intracranial sinuses, for the superior ophthalmic vein receives blood from the facial vein. Further input into the front of the cavernous sinus comes from a sinus running along the lesser wing of the sphenoid, called the 'sphenoparietal sinus'. Superficial middle cerebral and some inferior cerebral veins also drain into the cavernous sinus. The two cavernous sinuses communicate with each other around the pituitary stalk by anterior and posterior intercavernous sinuses. Most of the blood is drained from the cavernous sinus by the superior and inferior petrosal sinuses. The superior petrosal sinus transfers blood to the transverse sinus while the inferior petrosal sinus takes blood to the internal jugular vein. Blood also travels to the pterygoid venous plexus from the cavernous sinus by veins which pass through the foramen ovale, the foramen lacerum, and the foramen of Vesalius. The posterior ends of the cavernous sinus are also united over the clivus by means of a basilar plexus of veins. At the back of the foramen magnum is a small occipital sinus in the free edge of the falx cerebelli. Basilar and occipital sinuses communicate with the vertebral venous plexuses. Not all blood therefore leaves the skull by the internal jugular vein, some leaves by means of these communications to reach the vertebral plexuses.

THE INTRACRANIAL COURSE OF THE INTERNAL CAROTID AND VERTEBRAL ARTERIES

1. The internal carotid artery

The internal carotid and the vertebral arteries enter the cranial cavity to supply the brain. The internal carotid artery ascends through the carotid foramen in the petrous temporal bone, and then curves forwards and medially through the carotid canal. The walls of the canal separate it from the middle ear and the auditory tube. Indeed, in the infant the bone between these structures is particularly thin and often contains perforations. The trigeminal ganglion is also close to the artery, for it sits on the upper surface of the petrous apex above the roof of the canal. When the artery emerges from the front of the canal it lies in the middle cranial fossa above the fibrocartilaginous plug which fills the foramen lacerum. It then continues to the side of the body of the sphenoid and runs through the cavernous sinus. Near the front of the sinus, it curves upwards to gain the medial side of the anterior clinoid process. Here it pierces the dura of the roof of the cavernous sinus. The artery now turns back, passes below the optic nerve, then between the optic and oculomotor nerves, and terminates at the medial end of the lateral sulcus as anterior and middle cerebral arteries (Figs. 2.7, 3.9).

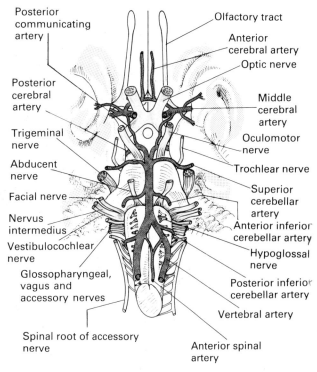

Fig. 2.7 The base of the brain — cranial nerves and arteries

While in the carotid canal the internal carotid artery gives minute twigs to the ear. In the cavernous sinus it gives branches to the trigeminal ganglion and to the surrounding meninges. It also gives inferior and superior hypophysial arteries to supply the pituitary (Fig. 2.8). The inferior arteries form an anastomotic ring around the posterior lobe of the pituitary. The superior artery supplies branches to the hypothalamus and the infundibulum, and those branches which end in the infundibulum terminate as small capillary tufts. From these, long portal vessels descend to supply the anterior lobe of the pituitary. Short portal vessels arise near the lower part of the infundibulum and also supply the anterior lobe. The portal vessels carry hormone releasing factors which control the secretory cells of the anterior lobe. During the course through the carotid canal and cavernous sinus, the carotid artery is surrounded by a plexus of sympathetic nerves and a minute plexus of veins. Once the carotid artery has pierced the roof

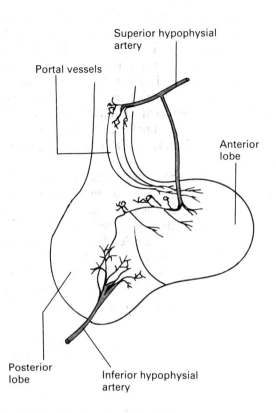

Superior hypophysial artery

Portal vessels

Anterior lobe

Posterior lobe

Inferior hypophysial artery

Fig. 2.8 The blood supply of the pituitary

of the cavernous sinus it gives the ophthalmic artery which enters the orbit through the optic canal.

The anterior cerebral artery is the smaller of the two terminal branches. It passes medially above the optic nerve to gain the longitudinal fissure between the two frontal lobes. The arteries are joined together by a short trunk called the 'anterior communicating artery'. The two anterior cerebral arteries curve around the genu of the corpus callosum and run back along its upper surface. Near the back of the corpus they anastomose with the posterior cerebral arteries. The middle cerebral artery is usually larger than the anterior, and runs in the lateral sulcus.

2. The vertebral artery

The vertebral artery, after piercing the dura and arachnoid in the cervical part of the vertebral column, ascends to the foramen magnum. In this pos-

ition it is anterior to the ascending rootlets of the spinal part of the accessory nerve. It ascends through the foramen magnum in front of the roots of the hypoglossal nerve, and unites with its partner of the opposite side at the lower border of the pons to form the basilar artery (Figs. 2.7, 2.17). Near its termination it gives an anterior spinal artery which descends through the foramen magnum to supply the spinal cord. The posterior inferior cerebellar artery is the largest branch of the vertebral artery, and gives a posterior spinal artery which also descends to the spinal cord. This artery, however, may arise from the vertebral artery itself. The basilar artery is found in a groove on the surface of the pons, within the pontine cistern. The branches of the basilar artery include an anterior inferior cerebellar artery, a superior cerebellar artery and a labyrinthine branch. This latter vessel enters the internal acoustic meatus. The terminal branches of the basilar artery are posterior cerebral arteries, each of which receives a posterior communicating branch from the corresponding internal carotid artery. A polygonal anastomosis is thus formed around the base of the brain enclosing the optic chiasma and contained within the interpeduncular cistern. The anastomosis, the circulus arteriosus of Willis, is formed in front by the two anterior cerebral arteries joined by the anterior communicating trunk, and behind by the posterior communicating arteries and posterior cerebral vessels. The anterior cerebral, middle cerebral, and posterior communicating arteries are all closely attached to the brain by means of small perforating branches.

3. Cerebral angiography

Contrast medium may be injected directly into both carotid and vertebral arteries in the neck by percutaneous injection. Although the carotid artery is fairly easy to enter by this method, the vertebral artery is more difficult to localise, and the procedure is often painful. The method of choice is to use the Seldinger technique, by which a catheter is introduced through a femoral artery under light sedation and local anaesthetic. Once the artery has been entered by the trocar, a guide wire is inserted into the lumen. The trocar is removed leaving a guide wire leading to the lumen of the femoral artery. The wire is used as a guide to feed a cannula into the artery, and is then withdrawn. The cannula is advanced along the aorta to the aortic arch where, under screen control, it can be made to enter any of the branches of the aorta. Both carotid and both vertebral arteries can thus be outlined by this single procedure (Fig. 2.9). The vessels and their major branches should be filmed in both lateral and frontal projections. Oblique and axial views, however, are also taken to show parts of the carotid tree in detail. Subtraction angiography is often performed to enhance the information on the angiogram. In principle, this technique demonstrates the difference between two radiographs, one made before and one after contrast medium has been injected.

Such pictures are available instantly with the aid of digital video and storage facilities. With the subtraction technique, many superimposed structures, a nuisance on the straight angiogram, are almost eliminated. Using this technique it is possible to take a satisfactory angiogram with only a small amount of contrast medium in the vessel. This can be acheived by a simple intravenous administration of medium, so avoiding intrarterial puncture.

On the lateral film the internal carotid artery may be located below the petrous temporal bone, but as it passes through the carotid canal it is largely lost in the shadow of the bone (Figs. 2.10, 2.11). Its ascent to the side of the sphenoid and through the cavernous sinus may then be followed. It takes a bend to reach the anterior clinoid process. This S-shaped curve of the intracavernous and supracavernous portions of the artery is called

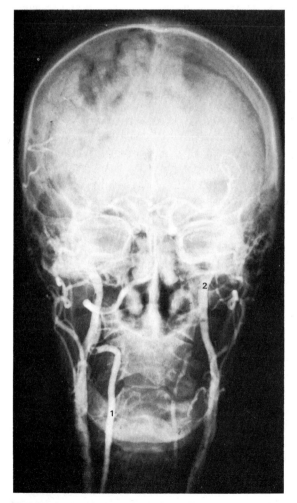

Fig. 2.9 A carotid and vertebral artery angiogram. 1: Vertebral artery. 2: Internal carotid artery.

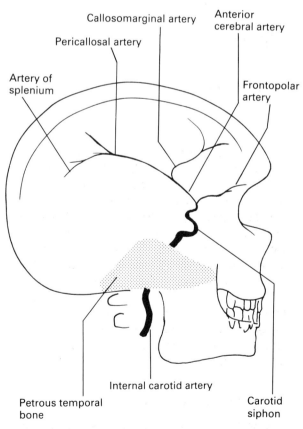

Fig. 2.10 A tracing of a carotid artery angiogram

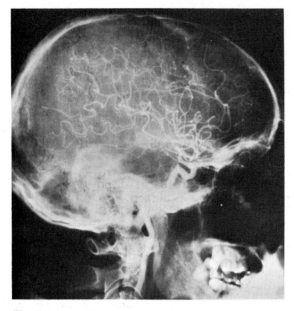

Fig. 2.11 A carotid artery angiogram — lateral view

syphon is foreshortened, but the T-shaped division of the internal carotid into anterior and middle cerebral branches is clear (Fig. 2.12). The anterior cerebral artery is located in the midline and callosomarginal and frontal polar branches may again be identified. The middle cerebral artery passes laterally from the T-shaped junction, and the first branches that are visible are the striate vessels. One artery in this group is usually larger than the others, and was termed by Charcot the 'artery of cerebral haemorrhage'. The parietal and temporal branches are foreshortened.

The vertebral artery, as it is traced through the upper part of the cervical column, curls out laterally in a wide loop from the foramen transversarium of the axis to that of the atlas (Fig. 2.13). It then proceeds towards the midline, piercing dura and arachnoid to enter the region of the foramen magnum. Here it may be traced up to the formation of the basilar artery, and its terminal posterior cerebral branches.

the carotid 'siphon'. It is an important part of the angiogram to inspect, for masses in the pituitary region will open out the curl in the artery. The ophthalmic branch may be traced forwards from the carotid artery in this region. An anterior choroidal branch and a posterior communicating branch also leave the carotid artery in this part of its course, and pass backwards. In a certain number of subjects the posterior cerebral artery fills during a carotid angiogram. After piercing the dura, the carotid divides into its two terminal branches, the anterior and middle cerebral arteries. The anterior cerebral artery, usually smaller than the middle, ascends between the two frontal lobes giving a branch which can be followed to the front pole of the frontal lobes. The main trunk of the anterior cerebral artery can be seen curving over the corpus callosum. A callosomarginal branch runs at a higher level over the roof of the lateral ventricle. On the lateral view, the middle cerebral artery is foreshortened, for its course takes it laterally to the lateral cerebral sulcus. Usually, several frontal, parietal, and temporal branches can be identified passing to the corresponding lobes of the brain.

On the frontal and oblique views, the carotid

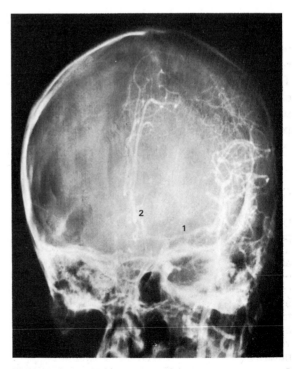

Fig. 2.12 A carotid artery angiogram — frontal view.
1: Middle cerebral. 2: Anterior cerebral.

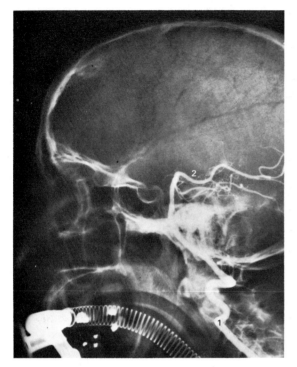

Fig. 2.13 A vertebral artery angiogram. 1: Vertebral artery. 2: Posterior cerebral artery.

in the temporal areas of the visual fields. There was evidence of a 6th cranial nerve lesion on the right, so that he could not direct the gaze far laterally with this eye. There was no neck rigidity.

This history suggested pressure in the region of the optic chiasma, also affecting the right 6th cranial nerve. The headache raised the possibility of a subarachnoid haemorrhage, and Digby was admitted for further investigation. A radiograph of his skull was normal. A lumbar puncture revealed normal CSF. An enhanced CT scan showed a large arteriovenous malformation in the region of the pituitary fossa (Fig. 2.14). Vascular aneurysms and malformations may occur at any point on the circle of Willis, but 90–95% of saccular aneurysms occur in the anterior part of the circle. Such aneurysms may rupture in adult life, and give rise to a subarachnoid haemorrhage. This produces severe headache, neck rigidity and a blood-stained CSF. After initial treatment, and localisation of the aneurysm by CT scan, the treatment usually involves tying the neck of the aneurysm, or extracranial ligation of the carotid. Unfortunately Digby had a large arteriovenous malformation, which would be very difficult to treat surgically. 3 days after admission he suffered a severe subarachnoid haemorrhage, and died 24 hours later.

During the venous phase of contrast radiography, the lateral film will give a picture of the superior sagittal sinus and the transverse sinus. The internal cerebral veins and great cerebral vein of Galen may be identified as they enter the straight sinus, and near the internal occipital protuberance the confluence of sinuses will be outlined.

CASE 4

Digby Davenport, a 24-year-old stockbroker, experienced a sudden, severe frontal headache during an argument with a client. He was nauseated, and later vomited twice. When seen in the emergency unit, the headache was worse, and generalised. He was lucid. On close questioning, he admitted that he had suffered repeated headaches for several months, and had noticed some blurring of vision. He also experienced occasional double vision, but insisted that this was intermittent in nature. Examination revealed a normal pulse and blood pressure. Initial neurological examination indicated that he had loss of vision in both eyes

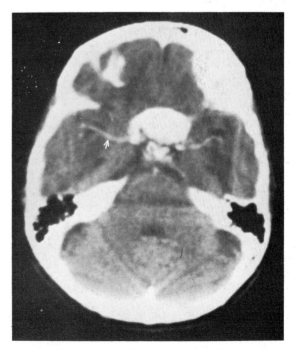

Fig. 2.14 Digby Davenport. CT scan of the head. The white arrow points to the middle cerebral artery.

CASE 5

Veronica Dooley, a 63-year-old cinema attendant, experienced a sudden and severe attack of dizziness after work. She was driven home by a friend, but on arrival was unable to stand. She vomited several times. She was unable to sleep, and was seen by her family physician early the following morning. He thought that she could be suffering from an infection in the inner ear (vestibulitis), and arranged her admission to hospital. She was seen by the neurologist, who thought that the clinical picture could have been produced by blockage of the vertebral artery or posterior inferior cerebellar artery. In this condition, the lateral medulla is deprived of blood, and a syndrome of sudden dizziness, nausea, vomiting, ataxia and nystagmus ensues.

Veronica's vertebral artery angiogram showed occlusion of the left vertebral artery (Fig. 2.15). She was admitted for investigation and treatment. The results of vertebral artery occlusion vary considerably, and depend on the relative size of the vertebral arteries and the point of blockage. Occasionally, inadequate vertebral artery flow is the result of a problem in the subclavian artery. If the subclavian artery is blocked proximal to the origin of a vertebral artery, exercise of the arm on that side draws blood from the vertebral system into the arm. This produces symptoms of vertebral artery insufficiency, and has therefore been called the 'subclavian steal' syndrome. Veronica had a CT scan which showed a meningioma compressing the vertebral artery. This was removed surgically. She made a good recovery, but was left with residual ataxia.

THE CRANIAL NERVE POSITIONS IN THE CRANIAL CAVITY

The olfactory bulbs and tracts are found in the anterior cranial fossa. The olfactory nerves themselves arise from bipolar cells in the nasal mucous membrane and pass through the cribriform plate of the ethmoid to enter the inferior surface of the bulbs. Very rarely a defect may occur in the ethmoid in this position, which allows a small diverticulum of meninges to protrude beneath the nasal mucous membrane. Rupture gives rise to spontaneous rhinorrhea. A meningocele may also be found in this situation on rare occasions. The optic nerves are located in the middle cranial fossa. Each nerve, surrounded by meninges, emerges from its optic canal and joins its fellow in the optic chiasma. From here the optic tracts diverge as they pass towards the brain. The optic nerves and tracts have important vascular relationships (Figs. 2.7, 3.9). The internal carotid artery, having emerged from the cavernous sinus, occupies the angle between the optic nerve and the optic tract, and here gives off its middle and anterior cerebral branches. The middle cerebral artery continues posterolateral to the optic nerve and is here held against the anterior perforated substance by many small branches. It then disappears from view in the depths of the lateral fissure. The anterior cerebral artery crosses above the optic nerve and then between the bases of the olfactory tracts before disappearing between the two cerebral hemispheres. The posterior communicating artery, a branch of the internal carotid, passes back below the optic tract. The ophthalmic artery lies in close relationship with the inferior surface of the optic nerve. The optic nerves and the circle of Willis are contained in the chiasmatic cistern of CSF.

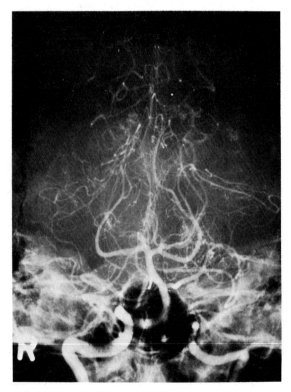

Fig. 2.15 Veronica Dooley. Vertebral artery angiogram.

The three motor nerves to the muscles of the orbit traverse the cavernous sinus to reach the superior orbital fissure (Fig. 2.16). The oculomotor and trochlear nerves pierce the roof of the cavernous sinus just medial to the free border of the tentorium as it approaches the anterior clinoid process. Close to its origin, the oculomotor nerve squeezes between the posterior cerebral and the superior cerebellar arteries (Fig. 2.7). It crosses the ridge formed by the attached margin of the tentorium and reaches the roof of the cavernous sinus. This margin, it will be recalled, is attached to the posterior clinoid process, and the nerve may be compressed on this edge if there is an increase in intracranial pressure. Once through the roof, the oculomotor nerve runs in the lateral wall of the sinus to reach the superior orbital fissure. The trochlear nerve also travels through the lateral wall of the cavernous sinus on its way to the superior orbital fissure. The abducent nerve approaches the dura in the posterior cranial fossa in close association with the anterior inferior cerebellar artery. It pierces the dura of the inferior petrosal sinus and enters the cavity of the cavernous sinus. In so doing, it usually passes below a fibrous band which binds the apex of the petrous temporal bone to the side of the pituitary fossa — the petroclinoid ligament of Gruber. As it passes through the cavernous sinus, the 6th nerve lies below and lateral to the internal carotid artery.

With the exception of the optic nerve, the trigeminal nerve is the largest of the cranial nerves. It arises from the pons by means of two roots — a large sensory and a small motor root. The nerve approaches the dura covering the posterior slope of the petrous temporal bone. Here, near the ridge, the nerve pushes the dura under the superior petrosal sinus and carries it deep to the dural floor of the middle cranial fossa. This produces a dural cave, the trigeminal or Meckel's cave, beneath the dura of the middle cranial fossa, with the opening to the cave in the posterior fossa. The sensory ganglion of the trigeminal nerve lies in the cave near the apex of the petrous temporal bone. Its official name is now the 'trigeminal ganglion', but in the past it has had other names such as the 'semilunar' or 'Gasserian' ganglion. A depression made by the ganglion on the apex of the petrous temporal bone can be found in most skulls. The

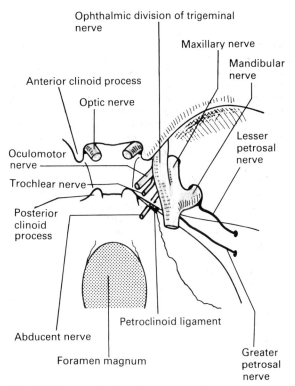

Fig. 2.16 Nerves related to the cavernous sinus

Labels: Ophthalmic division of trigeminal nerve; Maxillary nerve; Mandibular nerve; Anterior clinoid process; Optic nerve; Lesser petrosal nerve; Oculomotor nerve; Trochlear nerve; Posterior clinoid process; Petroclinoid ligament; Abducent nerve; Foramen magnum; Greater petrosal nerve

evaginated posterior fossa dura fuses with the peripheral part of the trigeminal ganglion, but a variable amount of the posterior half of the trigeminal ganglion is bathed in CSF. The subarachnoid space is more extensive on the deep surface of the ganglion and almost extends to the mandibular division. Three branches lead from the trigeminal ganglion — the ophthalmic, maxillary and mandibular divisions. The ophthalmic and maxillary divisions run in the lateral wall of the cavernous sinus, the ophthalmic division going to the superior orbital fissure, and the maxillary to the foramen rotundum. The mandibular division passes directly to the foramen ovale. The motor root of the trigeminal nerve lies deep to the trigeminal ganglion as it passes through the cave, and leaves the skull with the mandibular division.

The facial and vestibulocochlear nerves lie close together as they pass across the subarachnoid space to the internal acoustic meatus (Fig. 2.17). The facial nerve has a motor root and a root called the 'nervus intermedius' or 'sensory' root. The 8th nerve lies to the lateral side of the nervus intermedius. Indeed, until it reaches the internal acoustic meatus, the nervus intermedius is often fused with the 8th nerve rather than with the 7th. Within the meatus the motor root of the 7th nerve lies on the upper and anterior surface of the vestibulocochlear nerve grooving its surface. The nervus intermedius lies between them. The course of the anterior inferior cerebellar artery takes it ventral to the 7th and 8th nerves as well as to the abducens. Indeed, it often forms a small loop which travels for a short distance with the 7th and 8th nerves into the internal acoustic meatus before emerging for distribution to the cerebellum. The labyrinthine branch of the basilar artery (or of the anterior inferior cerebellar artery) accompanies the 7th and 8th nerves into the meatus.

The glossopharyngeal, vagus and accessory nerves leave the skull through the jugular foramen. This foramen is divided by fibrous septa into three compartments — anterior, middle and posterior. The anterior compartment transmits the inferior petrosal sinus. (A meningeal branch of the ascending pharyngeal artery also enters the skull by this route.) The posterior compartment is large, and transmits the sigmoid sinus. (A meningeal branch of the occipital artery enters the skull through this compartment.) The 9th, 10th and 11th cranial nerves use the middle compartment. The three nerves are closely related to the posterior inferior

cerebellar artery (Fig. 2.7). The glossopharyngeal nerve leaves the skull through the pyramidal notch in the petrous temporal side of the jugular foramen. Occasionally, there is a bony canal for the nerve. The nerve carries its own sheath of dura as it leaves the cranial cavity. The accessory nerve has two portions, a spinal part and a cranial part. The spinal part of the nerve arises by a series of rootlets from the upper five segments of the cervical part of the spinal cord. On emerging from the cord they form a trunk which ascends between the ligamentum denticulatum and the dorsal roots of the upper spinal nerves. The trunk enters the skull through the foramen magnum behind the vertebral artery (Fig. 2.17). The spinal root joins the cranial root for a short distance, but soon separates as the nerve passes through the jugular foramen. The cranial root is destined to join the vagus just below the jugular foramen, and is distributed with certain branches of the vagus nerve. The hypoglossal nerve is closely related to the vertebral artery near the foramen magnum and leaves the skull through the hypoglossal, or anterior condylar, canal.

CASES 1, 2 AND 3 (CONCLUDED)

Tom
The stories of Tom, Dick and Harry have been followed through Chapters 1 and 2. Tom did not sur-

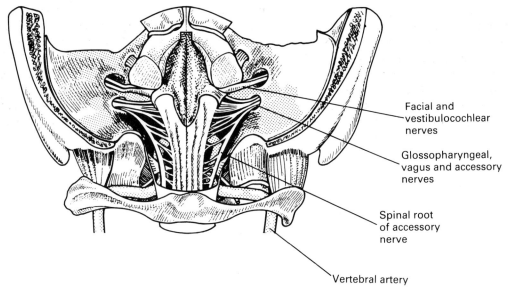

Facial and vestibulocochlear nerves

Glossopharyngeal, vagus and accessory nerves

Spinal root of accessory nerve

Vertebral artery

Fig. 2.17 The cranial nerves in the posterior cranial fossa. The vertebral artery can be seen in front of the spinal accessory roots.

vive. He failed to regain consciousness, and died 2 days after the craniotomy. At autopsy he was found to have widespread cerebral damage and oedema.

Dick

Dick was discharged from hospital after 3 days of observations. He did not, however, return to work. His appetite was poor, he lost weight, and felt unwell. 8 weeks after the accident his condition worsened. He found it difficult to concentrate, and complained of double vision. On examination he had ptosis and looked down and to the right with his right eye. His right pupil was dilated, and only contracted sluggishly when a light was shone into this eye. These general and localised problems suggested increased intracranial pressure and a 3rd cranial nerve lesion.

A computed tomogram showed a right-sided old extracerebral haematoma in the right frontal region (Fig. 2.18). Compare this picture with that of the recent haematoma in Figure 2.2. Dick had a chronic haematoma which had liquefied, and resulted in the radiolucent area on CT. At operation, a chronic subdural collection was evacuated. He made a good recovery.

Harry

Harry had no recurrence of rhinorrhoea, and was back at work 6 months after the injury.

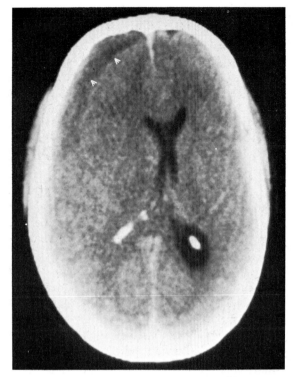

Fig. 2.18 Dick Duster. CT scan of the head. White arrows — edge of extracerebral collection of blood.

Head injuries are common. They are usually of minor severity, and cause no more than temporary inconvenience. The more severe head injuries, however, cause widespread cerebral damage and often have a fatal outcome. Between these two extremes the student will witness many grades. The initial assessment gives a baseline from which to follow the case, but should never be regarded as the final verdict. Complications may be heralded by subtle changes in the level of consciousness, and can occur at any time. The 'classical' story of a subdural haemorrhage, for example, is that there is a lucid interval of 24 hours or more after the injury, followed by deterioration. The medical student should not dwell on such preconceived patterns, but carefully conduct repeated neurological examinations on each patient under observation, and look critically at each radiograph and CT. In this way the student will find the care of head injury patients both interesting and rewarding.

3

THE ORBIT AND EYE

Facial injuries may involve the bones of the orbit, the surrounding air sinuses, the globe of the eye, or the nerves of the region. Tumours also occur in the orbit, or in adjacent parts of the maxillary air sinus, the nasopharynx, the nose or the cranial cavity. Although the fine details of the structure of the eye are the domain of the ophthalmologist, the student must be able to carry out an initial examination of the eye and its environment. This will require a knowledge of the bony orbit, the muscles and neurovascular structures associated with the eye, and the structure of the globe itself.

THE BONES OF THE ORBIT

The bony orbit contains and protects the eyeball. The roof of the orbit is formed mainly by the orbital plate of the frontal bone (Fig. 3.1). The bone forms a sharp supraorbital margin with a supraorbital notch. The frontal air sinus lies within the frontal bone above the medial half of this margin. A small trochlear fossa lies in the medial corner of the roof near the margin, and gives attachment to a fibrocartilaginous loop associated with the tendon of the superior oblique muscle. At the lateral extremity of the roof, again near the margin, is a lacrimal fossa which in life contains the orbital part of the lacrimal gland. At the back of the orbit, the frontal bone articulates with the lesser and greater wings of the sphenoid.

The floor of the orbit is formed mostly by the maxilla and the zygomatic bone. Towards the back of the orbit, the floor is separated from the greater

wing of the sphenoid by the inferior orbital fissure. A probe passed downwards through this fissure leads to the pterygopalatine fossa. A groove leading to the infraorbital canal in the maxilla, may be traced forwards from the inferior orbital fissure to the infraorbital foramen on the face. The lateral wall of the orbit is formed by the zygomatic bone in front and the greater wing of the sphenoid behind. Occasionally, however, the maxilla insinuates itself between the zygomatic bone and the greater wing of sphenoid to take a larger part in the formation of the orbital wall. Two minute canals will be found in the zygomatic bone close to

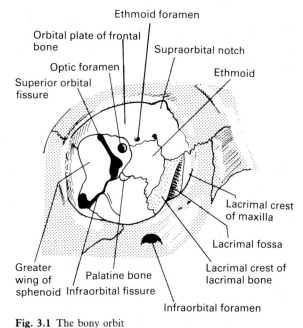

Fig. 3.1 The bony orbit

its union with the sphenoid. In life, these conduct the zygomaticofacial and zygomaticotemporal nerves from the inferior orbital fissure to the side of the face. The medial wall of the orbit is thin and composed of several bones. In front is the frontal process of the maxilla. This bears an anterior lacrimal crest which gives attachment to part of the orbicularis oculi muscle. Behind the crest, the maxilla and delicate lacrimal bone together form a lacrimal groove which houses the lacrimal sac. The groove is limited behind by the posterior lacrimal crest of the lacrimal bone itself. Lacrimal fibres of the orbicularis oculi are attached to this posterior crest. The lower end of the lacrimal bone presents a small hook-like hamulus. This partly surrounds the lower end of the lacrimal groove and leads to a nasolacrimal canal which in turn leads to the lateral wall of the nose. The orbital plate of the ethmoid lies behind the lacrimal bone in the medial wall of the orbit. This plate is particularly thin, and covers the ethmoidal air sinuses. Anterior and posterior foramina for ethmoidal nerves may be found within the suture between the ethmoid and the frontal bones. At the lower posterior corner of the ethmoid, a small segment of the orbital process of the palatine bone is exposed in the bony wall. Behind the ethmoid is the apex of the orbit formed by the body of the sphenoid and its optic canal. Below this is the superior orbital fissure between the lesser and greater wings of the sphenoid. The optic foramen, found in the body of the sphenoid, can be identified radiologically with an oblique view of the orbit (Fig. 3.2).

THE EXTRAOCULAR MUSCLES

Six muscles arise from the bony orbit, insert into the globe of the eye, and are responsible for the movements of the eyeball. A further muscle is found in the orbit, however, but it is an elevator of the upper eyelid.

The four recti arise from a fibrous ring called the 'common annular tendon' or the 'fibrous ring of Zinn' (Fig. 3.3). It encloses the optic canal and the medial end of the superior orbital fissure. The superior rectus arises from the upper part of the ring and the inferior rectus from the lower

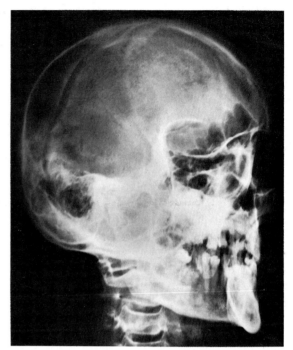

Fig. 3.2 Oblique radiograph of the skull

part. The medial rectus arises from the ring medial to the optic foramen and the lateral rectus from the lateral side of the ring as it straddles the superior orbital fissure. A small extra head of origin of the lateral rectus arises separately from the greater wing of the sphenoid. Each rectus passes forwards to insert into the eyeball in front of its equator. The recti, despite their name, do not lie straight in the sagittal plane when the eye looks directly ahead in its 'primary' position (Fig. 3.4). Neither the orbital axis nor the recti align themselves with this visual axis. The medial walls of the two orbits are parallel with each other, but the lateral walls are not, for they make an angle of 90° with each other. The midline of the triangular orbit is called the 'axis of the orbit', and makes an angle of 23° with the primary visual axis. The recti, arising near the apex of the triangle, are aligned with the axis of the orbit.

The superior and inferior oblique muscles effectively *pull* from the *front* of the roof and the floor of the orbit respectively. From here, they pass backwards to insert into the eyeball *behind* its

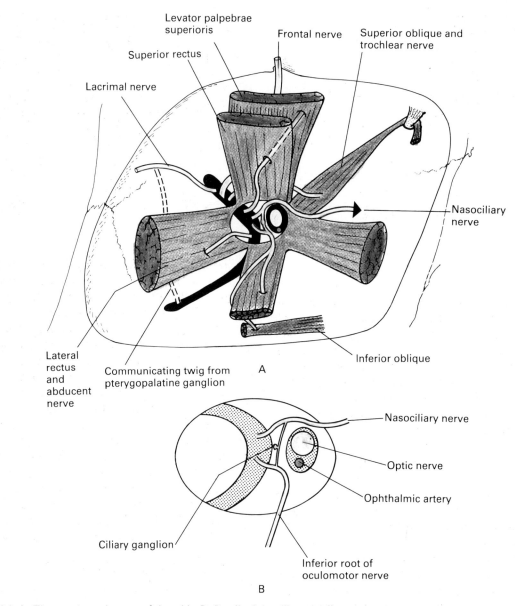

Fig. 3.3 A: The muscles and nerves of the orbit. B: Detail of the ciliary ganglion.

equator. The superior oblique in fact *arises* from the body of the sphenoid at the back of the orbit, but it passes to the roof of the orbit and gives way to a tendon which changes direction. The tendon does this by hooking through a pulley or 'trochlea'. The tendon then passes obliquely backwards beneath the superior rectus to insert into the eyeball. Its effective pull is thus from the trochlea. The inferior oblique arises from the maxilla in the floor of the orbit. It passes superficial to the inferior rectus insertion and then deep to the lateral rectus to reach the eyeball behind the equator. The pull of the obliques, like that of the recti, is also related to the axis of the orbit. Unlike the recti, however, their pull is set at right angles to the axis.

For the sake of simplicity the movements of the eyeball are defined as 'elevation' when the pupil is directed upwards and 'depression' when the

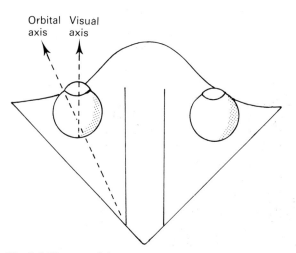

Fig. 3.4 The axes of the eye

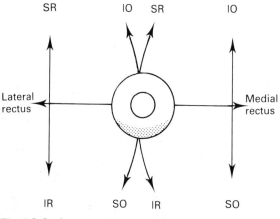

Fig. 3.5 Ocular movements

pupil is directed downwards. 'Adduction' describes the pupil looking medially and 'abduction' looking laterally. There are further movements, however, for if the head is tilted relative to the body, reflex torsional movements occur around the visual axis. Inward rotation or 'intorsion' is a movement which would cause an object placed on the top of the eyeball to fall over towards the nose. The opposite movement is external rotation or 'extorsion'. Movements of the medial and lateral recti are fairly easy to understand; the medial rectus adducts the eyeball and the lateral rectus abducts it. On the other hand careful attention should be paid to the movements produced by the superior and inferior recti and obliques. The *chief* actions of the superior and inferior recti are to elevate and depress the eyeball respectively. If, however, the eye looks straight ahead in its primary position, the superior and inferior recti will also tend to adduct the eyeball. The chief actions of the superior and inferior obliques, because they insert behind the visual axis, are to depress and elevate respectively. Both obliques, however, also have an additional action of abduction because of their orientation. The *additional tendencies* of adduction by the superior and inferior recti and abduction by the obliques tend to *counterbalance one another* when the muscles are used in elevation and depression of the eyeball from the primary position (Fig. 3.5).

Consider depression of the eyeball in more de-

tail. Two muscles perform depression as a primary action, the inferior rectus and the superior oblique. It has been noted that when the eyeball looks directly downwards *from the primary position*, both muscles are used. The *adducting tendency* of the rectus is balanced by the *abducting tendency* of the oblique. It would thus be misleading to describe the 'function' of the superior oblique as turning the eye down 'and out', for the 'and out' effect is counterbalanced by the inferior rectus during normal eye movements. When, however, the lateral rectus moves the eye into extreme abduction, the inferior rectus lies in its optimal orientation to act as a depressor (Fig. 3.6). In this position the superior oblique has virtually no ability to depress, but can only produce intorsion if it contracts. On the other hand, when the medial rectus directs the gaze as far nasally as possible,

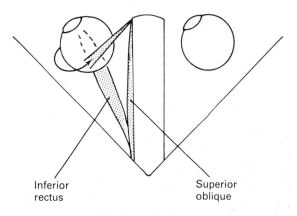

Fig. 3.6 Action of the superior oblique and inferior rectus on an abducted eye

it is the superior oblique's turn to be perfectly aligned to act as the prime depressor (Fig. 3.7). The inferior rectus is now ineffective, and is only capable of producing torsion. When considering the actions of the obliques and the superior and inferior recti, therefore, they must be tested in the direction of their strongest movements (Fig. 3.5).

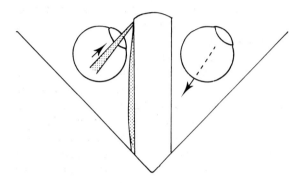

Fig. 3.7 Action of the superior oblique on an adducted eye

Clinically, therefore, to test the superior and inferior recti the patient must be asked to turn the eye as far laterally as possible and then be instructed to look upwards and downwards. This tests the superior and inferior recti respectively. The subject is then asked to turn the eye as far nasally as possible and to look up and down once again. This tests the inferior and superior obliques respectively. From this account it can be deduced that if there is a lesion causing paralysis of the superior oblique, the patient will be unable to look down when the eye is directed nasally. The subject can look laterally and downwards with lateral and inferior recti without any problem. Accounts which describe the action of the superior oblique as making the eye look 'down and out' serve only to confuse the student when testing normal function and describing abnormalities found in nerve lesions. In summary, the superior oblique turns the eye *down*, with a tendency to turn it out. The 'out' tendency, is usually counteracted by the inferior rectus. The most effective position for the superior oblique to act as a depressor is with the eyeball fully adducted.

The levator palpebrae superioris is a triangular muscle which arises from the lesser wing of the sphenoid above the optic canal. It passes forwards above the superior rectus and fans out into a flat aponeurosis which splits into superior and inferior lamellae (Fig. 3.8). The fibres of the superior lamella pass through the orbicularis oculi muscle to the skin of the upper eyelid. A few fibres are attached to the front of the superior tarsus. The inferior lamella is smaller, and is attached to the upper margin of the tarsus. Fibres in this region are partly formed of non-striated muscle, called the 'muscle of Müller'. The rest of the levator is made of striated, voluntary muscle. The lamellae of the levator palpebrae superioris have lateral and medial horns. The lateral horn is particularly prominent, and grooves the lacrimal gland, dividing it into palpebral and orbital parts. At the medial side, the aponeurosis gains a further attachment to the medial palpebral ligament.

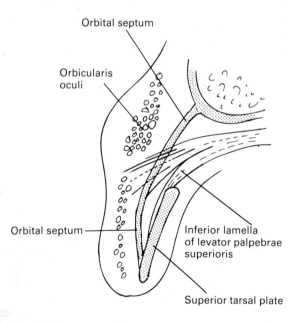

Fig. 3.8 The upper eyelid

NEUROVASCULAR STRUCTURES IN THE ORBIT

1. The optic nerve

The optic nerve fibres have glial and not Schwann

cell sheaths. This is because the nerves, together with the retina, are really extensions of the brain. Almost all of the fibres in the optic nerve are afferent, and arise in the ganglionic layer of the retina. There are a few efferent fibres, but their function is unknown. The optic nerve is enclosed throughout its length by sheaths of dura, arachnoid and pia. The three sheaths, including the subarachnoid space, are continuous with those of the brain, and extend as far as the eyeball. Septa from the pia subdivide the optic nerve into fascicles. The fibres of the nerve converge on the optic disc, 3 mm to the nasal side of the centre of the back of the eyeball. At the disc the fibres pierce the choroid and the lamina cribrosa of the sclera.

Traced from the eyeball, the optic nerve runs a sinuous course backwards and medially to the optic canal. At the back of the orbit it is intimately surrounded by the four recti as they arise from the fibrous ring (Fig. 3.3). In the orbital part of its course the optic nerve is related to the ophthalmic artery. The artery lies below and lateral to the optic nerve in the optic canal, but crosses above it in the orbit, and continues towards the medial orbital wall. The central artery of the retina, a branch of the ophthalmic artery, pierces the inferior surface of the optic nerve within the orbit and passes in the nerve to the optic disc. The nasociliary nerve accompanies the ophthalmic artery above the optic nerve, and also travels towards the medial wall of the orbit. The nerve to the medial rectus passes below the optic nerve. On the lateral side of the optic nerve, between it and the lateral rectus, is a small parasympathetic ganglion, the ciliary ganglion.

Once through the optic canal, the optic nerve runs backwards and medially into the optic chiasma (Fig. 3.9). In this part of its course the nerve has the anterior cerebral artery above it, and the internal carotid artery on its lateral side. The optic chiasma itself rests on the diaphragma sellae, a short distance behind the optic groove. The chiasma is related to the infundibulum of the pituitary. The anterior communicating artery lies above it, and laterally is the internal carotid artery. The optic tracts carry the optic fibres from the posterolateral angles of the chiasma towards the interpeduncular fossa.

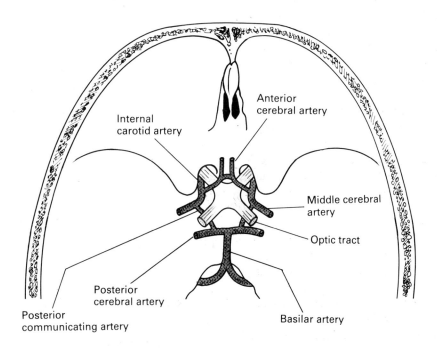

Fig. 3.9 The relations of the optic chiasma

Within the optic nerves the fibres from the upper and lower parts of the retina lie above and below respectively. Fibres from the temporal quadrants lie laterally, and those from the nasal quadrants, medially. Fibres from the macula occupy the lateral part of the nerve at first but then lie close to the medial margin near the optic chiasma. Here they form a flattened band which passes through the central region of the chiasma. In the chiasma, fibres from the nasal half of each retina cross to the optic tract of the opposite side. The macular fibre bundle lies above these decussating fibres. Fibres from the temporal half of the retina pass back into the optic tract of the same side. In the optic tracts the fibres from the macula become eccentric and occupy a dorsolateral position within the tract. Several fibre bundles have been described in the chiasma which are not derived from the optic nerve, but their origin and function are unknown. The optic nerve and chiasma are supplied by blood vessels which form a plexus in the pia. Contributions pass to this plexus from the internal carotid, superior hypophyseal, anterior cerebral, anterior communicating, ophthalmic and ciliary arteries.

CASE 1 (CONTINUED FROM CHAPTER 1, CASE 4)

Dotty Dobson's skull radiograph showed an enlarged pituitary fossa with a double floor (See Fig. 1.10). This indicated a possible expanding tumour in the pituitary fossa. The relationships of the pituitary fossa are important in such conditions, for expansion may cause pressure effects on any of the surrounding vital structures. On either side of the fossa is the cavernous sinus. Lateral expansion into a sinus may therefore cause pressure on the oculomotor, trochlear or abducent nerves or on the ophthalmic and maxillary divisions of the trigeminal nerve. The internal carotid artery is also in a close relationship to the pituitary fossa, both in the cavernous sinus and near its termination at the medial side of the anterior clinoid process. The optic nerves, chiasma, and tracts are particularly vulnerable, and Dotty had complained of problems of vision. Careful assessment of her fields of vision revealed that she had loss of vision in both temporal fields (bitemporal hemianopia). This could be explained by a lesion affecting the nasal fibres from each retina at the chiasma (Fig. 3.10). Such visual disturbances are important

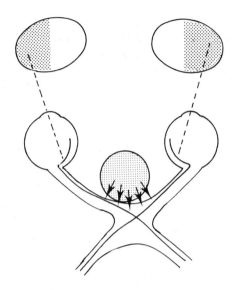

Fig. 3.10 Dotty Dobson. The effects of the tumour on the visual fields.

to recognise early, because it is often possible to save sight by surgical removal of the tumour. Dotty was sent for CT of the pituitary region.

2. The oculomotor, trochlear, and abducent nerves, and the ophthalmic branch of the trigeminal nerve

The course of these nerves through the cavernous sinus is described in Chapter 2. Within the cavernous sinus, the 3rd, 4th and 6th cranial nerves communicate with the ophthalmic division of the trigeminal nerve. They also communicate with the sympathetic fibres around the carotid artery. The nerves rearrange themselves as they pass towards the superior orbital fissure. Just before the fissure, the ophthalmic nerve divides into its three terminal branches — lacrimal, frontal and nasociliary nerves . The oculomotor, abducens and nasociliary nerves enter the orbit through the section of superior orbital fissure surrounded by the fibrous ring of Zinn. This brings them *within* the cone of muscles which surround the eyeball. The lacrimal, frontal and trochlear nerves, on the other hand, enter the orbit through the section of the fissure which is outside the fibrous ring. These three nerves therefore lie in the roof of the orbit above the cone of muscles. This upper part of the superior orbital fissure also transmits a meningeal branch of the lacrimal artery and an occasional branch from the middle meningeal artery. Rarely, this latter vessel may be large and even replace the ophthalmic artery as the main blood supply in the orbit.

a. The lacrimal, frontal and trochlear nerves

These three nerves lie outside the cone of muscles in the roof of the orbit (Fig. 3.3). The lacrimal nerve is a tiny branch of the ophthalmic division of the trigeminal nerve. As it approaches the lacrimal gland, it is joined by a twig of the zygomaticotemporal nerve or by a branch of the pterygopalatine ganglion itself. Either way, parasympathetic fibres from the ganglion pass through the inferior orbital fissure into the orbit. They are carried in the communicating twig up the lateral wall of the orbit to join the lacrimal nerve. Here, the parasympathetic fibres hitch-hike for a short distance before reaching the lacrimal gland, where they are secretomotor in function. The lacrimal nerve ends by supplying skin of the upper eyelid. The frontal nerve is a large, flat branch of the ophthalmic nerve, and is found above levator palpebrae superioris in the midline of the orbit. As it approaches the front of the orbit it divides into

supratrochlear and supraorbital branches. The supratrochlear branch emerges above the trochlea of the superior oblique, supplies branches to the upper eyelid and conjunctiva, and then ascends to the forehead where it pierces the frontalis and supplies skin on the front of the forehead. The supraorbital branch runs forwards through the supraorbital notch or foramen and also gives twigs to the upper eyelid and conjunctiva. It then pierces the frontalis to supply skin over the forehead and top of the head as far as the lambdoid suture. Both branches are accompanied by similarly named arteries. The trochlear nerve is also found outside the cone of muscles in the roof of the orbit. It is a small nerve, which after passing through the superior orbital fissure, soon enters the superior oblique muscle.

CASE 2

Neeten Chaudry, a 54-year-old farmer from one of the northern provinces of India, was first seen with an advanced tumour of the nasopharynx which had invaded the sphenoid air sinus, the maxilla and the medial wall of the left orbit (Fig. 3.11). On examination, there was blockage of the left nasal passage and mild proptosis of the left eye. He was unable to look down when the left eye was fully adducted. When asked to look in this direction he

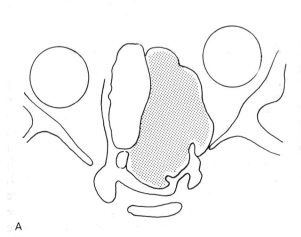

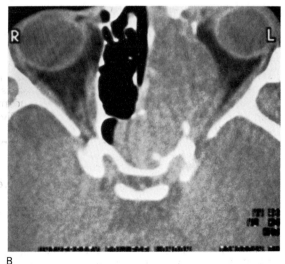

A   B

Fig. 3.11 Neeten Chaudry. A: Tracing of CT scan. B: CT scan of the head.

complained of double vision. These signs were indicative of a left 4th nerve lesion with paralysis of the superior oblique muscle. More careful examination also revealed rotational problems in the eye. The student will remember that the superior oblique helps in rotational movements of the eye as well as being a depressor. In spite of treatment, Neeten Chaudry died within 3 months of being seen.

b. The abducent, oculomotor and nasociliary nerves

These three nerves are found within the fibrous ring of Zinn and therefore lie within the cone of muscles at the back of the eyeball (see Fig. 3.3). The abducent nerve, after passing through the cav-

ernous sinus below and lateral to the internal carotid artery, passes through the superior orbital fissure and enters the orbital surface of the lateral rectus. The nasociliary nerve is a long branch of the ophthalmic division of the trigeminal nerve (Fig. 3.12). It travels towards the medial wall of the orbit, above the optic nerve, in company with the ophthalmic artery. Once at the medial wall it gives anterior and posterior ethmoidal branches and ends as the infratrochlear nerve. The anterior ethmoidal nerve ascends into the anterior cranial fossa through a small slit at the junction of ethmoid and frontal bones. Its course in the anterior cranial fossa is short, and it soon descends through a slit at the side of the crista galli. In this

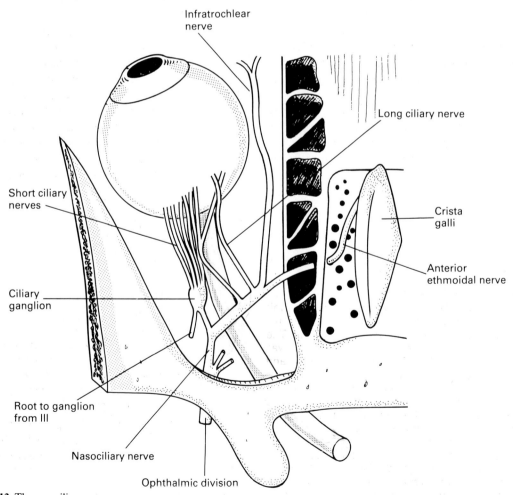

Fig. 3.12 The nasociliary nerve

way it reaches the nasal cavity where it gives internal nasal branches to the mucous membrane. It emerges as an external nasal branch to supply skin of the ala and vestibule of the nose. The posterior ethmoidal nerve is smaller and supplies fibres to ethmoidal and sphenoid air sinuses only. The infratrochlear branch leaves the orbit close to the pulley of the superior oblique. It supplies skin on the eyelids, the lacrimal caruncle and lacrimal sac. Two or three long ciliary nerves are given off from the nasociliary nerve as it passes over the optic nerve. These pierce the sclera and continue forwards between sclera and choroid for distribution to the ciliary body, iris and cornea. Just to the lateral side of the optic nerve, between it and the lateral rectus muscle, is the ciliary ganglion. The nasociliary nerve contributes a branch to this ganglion. Indeed, it appears as though the ganglion is suspended from the nasociliary nerve.

The oculomotor nerve, as it passes through the superior orbital fissure, divides into superior and inferior branches (see Fig. 3.3). The superior branch ascends on the lateral side of the optic nerve and supplies the superior rectus. After piercing this, it supplies levator palpebrae superioris; the involuntary fibres are supplied by sympathetic nerves. The inferior ramus runs below the optic nerve to supply the medial rectus. It also supplies a branch to the inferior oblique. A root enters the ciliary ganglion from this inferior oblique branch.

CASE 3

Vernon Smart, a 25-year-old tennis instructor, noticed occasional double vision while working. During the next 3 months this became considerably worse, and when seen at the ophthalmology unit he had an abducted left eye (lateral strabismus). There was also medial rotation of the eyeball. The upper left eyelid drooped (ptosis) and there was loss of accommodation. The pupil was dilated, and there was lack of constriction when a light was shone into the eye. The clinical picture was one of oculomotor nerve palsy. The extraocular muscles were paralysed with the exception of the lateral rectus and superior oblique. The lateral rectus held the eye in the abducted position, and with this direction of gaze the superior oblique medially rotated the globe (see Fig. 3.6). Paralysis of levator palpebrae superioris gave rise to ptosis, and of the ciliary muscle to loss of accommodation. The con-

strictor pupillae denervation resulted in a dilated pupil. Vernon was sent for a CT scan.

c. The ciliary ganglion

The ciliary ganglion is one of the four parasympathetic ganglia found in the head, and is concerned with the supply of the sphincter of the pupil and the ciliary muscle. Of the other three ganglia, the otic ganglion is concerned with secretomotor supply to the parotid gland, the pterygopalatine ganglion with secretion of the lacrimal gland and mucous glands in the nose and paranasal air sinuses, and the submandibular ganglion with the supply of salivary and mucous glands in the floor of the mouth. Each ganglion *lies close to one of the terminal branches of the trigeminal nerve* (Fig. 3.13). The ciliary ganglion lies close to the nasociliary nerve, the otic ganglion close to the mandibular nerve, the pterygopalatine ganglion close to the maxillary nerve, and the submandibular ganglion close to the lingual nerve. Parasympathetic fibres, however, do not reach the ganglia in the trigeminal nerve. They leave the brain stem through the oculomotor, facial, and glossopharyngeal nerves. (Parasympathetic outflow also leaves the brain in the vagus nerve, but this is not destined to supply the head.) Fibres from the 3rd nerve leave the branch to the inferior oblique to

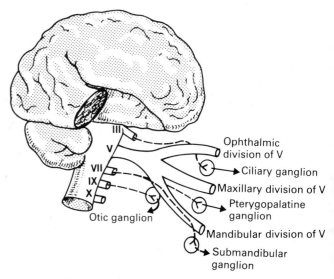

Fig. 3.13 Parasympathetic outflow from the brain

enter and synapse in the ciliary ganglion. Fibres from the 7th cranial nerve synapse in both the pterygopalatine ganglion and submandibular ganglion. Fibres from the 9th cranial nerve synapse in the otic ganglion. Apart from these parasympathetic fibres, other fibres pass through each of these ganglia without synapse. Sympathetic fibres reach the ciliary ganglion, for example, from the superior cervical sympathetic ganglion. These postganglionic fibres climb to the head through the internal carotid plexus of nerves, and pass through the ciliary ganglion without synapse to their target organ. Sensory fibres also pass through each of the head ganglia. They do not have their cell bodies in the parasympathetic ganglia, but in the sensory ganglion of the parent nerve or the trigeminal nerve. In the case of the otic ganglion, a few extra fibres traverse the ganglion; these are motor fibres to small striated muscles in the region.

The ciliary ganglion has a parasympathetic root from the inferior division of the oculomotor nerve, and a sympathetic root from the plexus around the internal carotid artery (Fig. 3.14). Only the para-

sympathetic fibres synapse in the ciliary ganglion. Both parasympathetic and sympathetic fibres are carried forwards to the eyeball in the short ciliary nerves, and sensory fibres from the cornea and eyeball pass in the reverse direction in these nerves. The sensory fibres enter the nasociliary nerve through its root to the ganglion, and travel along the trigeminal nerve. They have their cell bodies in the trigeminal ganglion. The sensory fibres bring back sensation from the cornea and eyeball. The parasympathetic supply is destined for the sphincter pupillae and ciliary muscle. The sympathetic supply entering the eye in the short ciliary nerves is vasoconstrictor in type for the vessels of the eyeball. Sympathetic fibres also reach the eyeball through the long ciliary branches of the nasociliary nerve, and pass to the dilator pupillae. Damage to the sympathetic trunk at the apex of the thoracic cavity or in the neck can damage the sympathetic supply to the eye. Horner's syndrome results — a combination of constricted pupil (miosis), slight drooping of the eyelid (ptosis), an absence of sweating and dilated blood vessels on the affected side of the face.

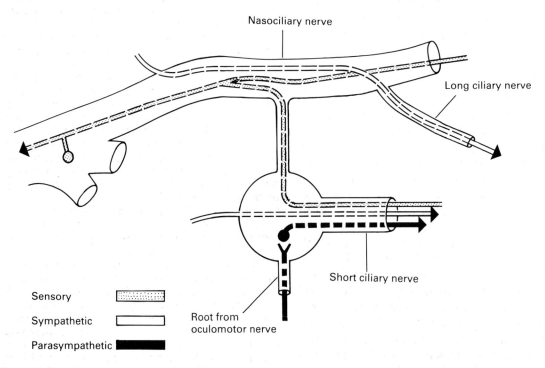

Fig. 3.14 The ciliary ganglion and its connections

SPECIAL INVESTIGATION OF THE PITUITARY REGION

Special attention should be paid to the region of the pituitary fossa in any radiographic examination of the skull. The size and shape of the fossa must be assessed, and the anterior and posterior clinoid processes inspected. The posterior clinoids and dorsum sellae are best seen in a view through the foramen magnum (see Fig. 1.16). Erosion of the boundaries of the fossa often indicates pressure from an adjacent mass. Sometimes the ligament of Grüber is calcified, and visible as a line behind and parallel to the dorsum sellae on the lateral radiograph. Calcified bridges are also occasionally found between the anterior and posterior clinoids, or between anterior and middle clinoids. The thickness of the bone of the sella must be assessed, for if there is chronic increased intracranial pressure, the sella will appear enlarged, and the bone of the fossa markedly thinned. The fossa is related to several structures which may be identified by conventional radiology and other imaging techniques. Below the fossa is the sphenoid air sinus, and this is visible on a lateral film. It varies considerably in both size and shape from individual to individual. If a precise estimate of the size of the sinus is required, lateral and fronto-occipital tomograms may be used to build up a picture. The neurosurgeon sometimes needs such information before approaching the pituitary fossa surgically through the nose and sphenoid air sinus. The pituitary fossa is closely related to the optic canals and optic chiasma. The chiasma lies in the chiasmatic cistern above the pituitary fossa. The optic canals may be identified on special orbital views of the skull. Computed tomography, combined with other special methods, will give detailed information about the pituitary fossa itself, the chiasmatic cistern above it, and the circle of Willis. The optic nerves can also be visualised on the scan, and the pituitary fossa, clinoids and dorsum sellae can be inspected once again. A cut through the chiasmatic cistern will show a 'six-pointed star' effect. With contrast enhancement the arteries of the circle of Willis will outline this star shape. The cistern itself may be outlined by positive contrast cisternography, contrast medium being injected into the subarachnoid space by either lumbar or suboccipital

puncture. A non-ionic contrast medium such as metrizamide is used for this investigation, and CT cuts will show the chiasmatic star with the optic nerves and pituitary stalk as filling defects within the star. The cavernous sinus lies on either side of the pituitary fossa, and this may be outlined by cavernous sinography. This procedure, rarely done nowadays, involves the insertion of a cannula into the frontal vein in the midline of the forehead. The facial veins are then compressed by means of pads held against the cheeks, and the contrast medium injected. The internal carotid arteries also lie on either side of the pituitary, and these may be outlined by angiography.

CASES 1 AND 2 (CONTINUED)

The CT of Dotty Dobson showed a large tumour in the pituitary region after enhancement (Fig. 3.15). After completion of investigations, Dotty was prepared for surgery.

Operation notes
The pituitary fossa was approached through the frontal region. After shaving the head, the scalp incision was made so that it would be largely concealed behind the hair-line (Fig. 3.16a). Several burr holes were made and a Gigli saw guide passed between the bone and dura from hole to hole (Fig. 3.16b). The bone between the lower two holes, however, was left uncut, and after gently prising, the bone flap was fractured. The flap thus had a pedicle of bone and temporalis muscle. This ensured a good blood supply to the flap when it was replaced. After opening the dura, the right frontal lobe was retracted. The right approach was preferred because the non-dominant right frontal lobe could be retracted without fear of producing dysphasia. The olfactory tract was identified on the under surface of the frontal lobe, and traced back to the optic tract and pituitary region. The large pituitary tumour with a suprasellar extension was removed. Dotty made a good recovery, and regained most of her eyesight.

If the problem had involved a small tumour, a trans-sphenoidal operation could have been performed. The pituitary fossa is approached through the sphenoid air sinus from the face, the tissue being removed with the aid of an operating microscope. Two routes are available for approaching the sphenoid air sinus — one through the roof of the nose and the other through the ethmoid air sinus. In the latter approach, a skin incision is

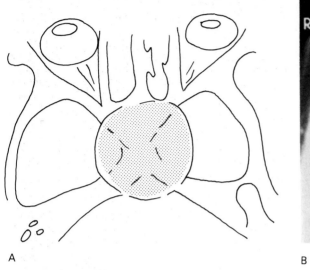

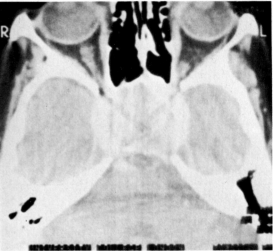

Fig. 3.15 Dotty Dobson. A: Tracing of CT scan. B: CT scan of head.

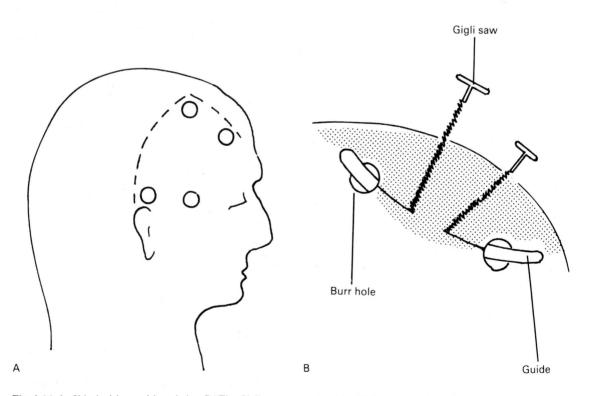

Fig. 3.16 A: Skin incision and burr holes. B: The Gigli saw.

made at the medial side of the orbit, and the ethmoid sinuses entered through the medial wall of the orbit. Further exploration takes the instrument through the sphenoid air sinus.

Vernon Smart's CT scan, with enhancement, showed a large tumour in the pituitary region (Fig. 3.17). The middle cerebral vessels were clearly outlined on the scan. Vernon was also taken for surgery, but died from complications in the early postoperative period.

THE FASCIAL SHEATH OF THE EYEBALL (THE CAPSULE OF TENON)

A thin fascial sheath covers the eyeball from the sclerocorneal junction in front to the optic nerve behind, and separates the eyeball from the orbital fat. The recti and obliques pierce the sheath before they gain insertion into the eyeball, and tubular extensions are reflected around each of these tendons (Fig. 3.18). The superior rectus sheath blends with the tendon of levator palpebrae superioris, while that of the inferior rectus blends with the sheath of the inferior oblique. Fascial expansions from the medial and lateral recti extend to the lacrimal and zygomatic bones respectively. These were called the 'check ligaments', because they were thought to check extremes of adduction and abduction. This is clearly not their function — they simply help in stabilising the eyeball during muscle pull. Beneath the eye the check ligaments are continuous with the sheath of the inferior rectus. A sling is formed in this way under the globe, called the 'suspensory ligament' of the eye.

The periosteum of the orbit or orbital fascia is loosely connected to the bone, and at the back of the eye is attached to the dural sheath of the optic nerve. In front, it is continuous with a membranous sheet, the orbital septum, which extends from the edge of the orbit into the upper and lower eyelids (See Fig. 3.8). The superficial lamella of the levator palpebrae superioris aponeurosis blends with the orbital fascia.

THE EYELIDS

The skin of the eyelids is thin, and there is little

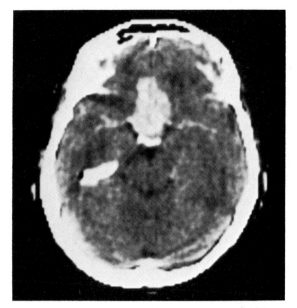

Fig. 3.17 Vernon Smart. Enhanced CT scan of the head.

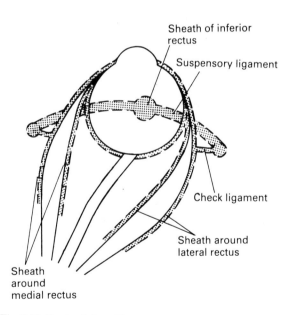

Fig. 3.18 Fascia of the orbit.

Labels: Sheath of inferior rectus; Suspensory ligament; Check ligament; Sheath around lateral rectus; Sheath around medial rectus

subcutaneous fat. Deep to the skin are the palpebral fibres of the orbicularis oculi muscle. Deep to this is a little loose areolar tissue which is continuous with the subaponeurotic layer of the scalp. Bleeding in this plane of the scalp will therefore track down into the upper eyelid. Support is given to the eyelids by fibrous tarsal plates. In the upper lid the superior lamella of the levator palpebrae aponeurosis is attached to the outer surface of the tarsus, and the inferior lamella to the edge of the tarsus. Both superior and inferior tarsi are attached to the orbital septum. The medial ends of the tarsal plates are attached to a strong ligament, the medial palpebral ligament, which in turn is anchored to the maxilla just in front of the anterior lacrimal crest. The lateral ends of the plates are attached to a lateral palpebral ligament which gains attachment to the zygomatic bone. The palpebral bundles of orbicularis oculi arise from both superficial and deep surfaces of the medial palpebral ligament. They sweep across the eyelids to insert as a lateral palpebral raphe *in front of* the lateral palpebral ligament. The fibres of the lacrimal part of the orbicularis oculi lie behind the lacrimal sac (see Ch. 12).

Tarsal glands (Meibomian glands) are embedded in the tarsi, and their ducts open on the free margins of the lid. They may be seen by everting the eyelids, when they appear as yellow streaks arranged in a row beneath the conjunctiva. They are, in fact, modified sebaceous glands. Their secretions spread over the margin of the eyelid and prevent tears from overflowing. The secretion may also form a film over the tears on the outer surface of the eye, so reducing evaporation. The innermost layer of the eyelid is the conjunctiva. This delicate membrane is reflected from the eyelids onto the eyeball at the superior and inferior fornices. On the eye, it covers the sclera and is continued as the corneal epithelium. A small lacrimal caruncle, composed of skin and containing sebaceous and sudoriferous glands is found in the medial angle of the eye. Just lateral to the caruncle is a fold of conjunctiva called the 'plica semilunaris'.

A foreign body often lodges under cover of the upper eyelid, and the lid must be everted during the search for the object. To do this, the eyelashes are grasped and the eyelid gently everted by folding it around an orange stick.

THE LACRIMAL APPARATUS

Tears are secreted by the lacrimal gland. This is located in the upper lateral part of the orbit. The lateral edge of the aponeurosis of the levator palpebrae superioris partly divides the gland into orbital and palpebral parts. The orbital part lies in the lacrimal fossa above the aponeurosis, and the smaller palpebral part lies below the aponeurosis within the upper eyelid. The ducts from the orbital part pass through the palpebral part and open into the superior fornix of the conjunctival sac. Many small accessory lacrimal glands are found near the conjunctival fornices. The parasympathetic secretomotor fibres for the lacrimal gland come from the facial nerve. Leaving the nerve as the greater superficial petrosal branch, they synapse in the pterygopalatine ganglion and travel in the zygomaticotemporal branch of the maxillary nerve to the orbit. Here a communicating branch takes them along the lateral wall of the orbit to their final path, the lacrimal nerve. They run a short distance in this latter nerve before entering the gland.

Tears sweep across the surface of the eye towards the medial angle. Here, on each eyelid, a punctum leads to a lacrimal canaliculus, which in turn enters the lacrimal sac. The superior canaliculus ascends at first, before passing down to the lacrimal sac. The sac lies in the lacrimal fossa between the anterior and posterior lacrimal crests. A layer of orbital fascia, the lacrimal fascia, separates the sac from the medial palpebral ligament in front, and from the lacrimal part of the orbicularis oculi behind. The nasolacrimal duct leads from the sac into the lateral wall of the nose. The bony canal for the duct is formed by the maxilla, lacrimal bone, and the inferior nasal concha. A small valve of mucous membrane is found in the duct near the nasal opening. The lacrimal apparatus may be examined radiologically by dacryocystography. Following instillation of local anaesthetic drops into the conjunctival sac, the lower punctum is dilated, and a tiny catheter inserted into the canaliculus. A small amount of an oily contrast medium is injected. The patient often complains of a bad taste at the back of the mouth because some of the medium has reached the nasopharynx.

RADIOLOGY OF THE ORBIT

The orbital walls and the optic canal may be visualised on special views of the head (see Fig. 3.2). For detailed examination of the orbital cavity and its contents, however, computed tomography is the examination of choice (Fig. 3.19). The optic nerve and recti are outlined on computed tomograms, together with details of the eyeball itself. Figure 3.20 is a CT of the orbits of a patient with Von Recklinhausen's disease (neurofibromatosis). In this condition tumours derived from the sheath of both peripheral and cranial nerves occur. The optic nerve has been involved on the left side, and is thicker than the nerve on the normal side. The lower picture in Figure 3.20 is a horizontal scan. The optic nerve tumour is the white mass at the apex of the left orbit. Note that the left eye has been pushed forwards by the tumour. The dotted line indicates the plane of the coronal section shown below in Figure 3.20. The recti and optic nerve are clearly shown on the section of the right eye, but the left optic nerve is grossly enlarged. The dotted line in Figure 3.21 shows the plane of

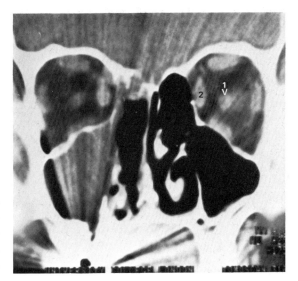

Fig. 3.19 CT scan of the orbits. 1: White arrow = optic nerve. 2: medial rectus.

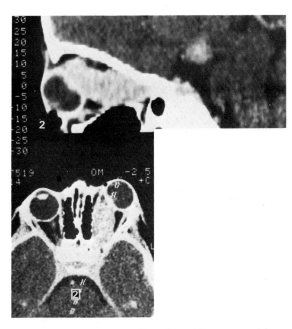

Fig. 3.20 Orbital CT scans of a patient with a tumour of the left optic nerve. See text for explanation. (By kind permission of Professor W. Ian McDonald, Institute of Neurology, The National Hospital, Queen Square, London.)

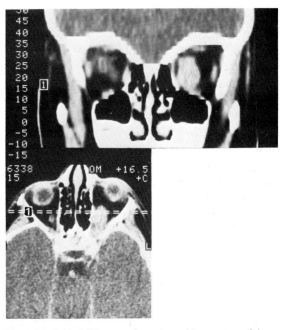

Fig. 3.21 Orbital CT scans of a patient with a tumour of the left optic nerve. See text for explanation. (By kind permission of Professor W. Ian McDonald, Institute of Neurology, The National Hospital, Queen Square, London.)

the sagittal section in the upper picture. This shows the size of the optic nerve tumour, and the protrusion of the eyeball. Magnetic resonance imaging (MRI) may also be used to outline orbital structures.

Radiology is often required to confirm the presence and position of a foreign body within the eyeball. Such foreign bodies are often metal fragments which fly off a hammer or other tool when it strikes a hard surface. These dangerous fragments travel at a high velocity, and easily penetrate the globe of the eye. If there is a history of using a hammer or similar tool in a case of eye injury, it is mandatory to proceed with radiology of the orbit. Metal splinters are for the most part opaque, but aluminium is not opaque. Glass splinters are often difficult to show radiologically. Once a foreign body has been confirmed, it must be accurately localised within the orbit by taking several radiographic views. A more accurate system, however, uses a Lo Vac Worst contact lens. This small plastic lens has a fine metal ring embedded in its periphery. It has a tiny central opening attached to a minute plastic tube, which in turn is connected to a small suction bulb. The eye is anaesthetised with local anaesthetic drops and the contact lens applied to the cornea. A little suction applied by means of the bulb will hold the lens firmly in place. Radiographs have the circular metal ring of the lens as an external reference, and this allows accurate localisation of the foreign body. If there has been a corneal laceration, however, this method is contraindicated.

THE EYEBALL

A detailed account of the structure of the eyeball is beyond the scope of this book. The medical student, however, should understand the basic structure of the globe of the eye and be able to perform an initial examination of the eye. Apart from the many common diseases and injuries afflicting the eye, the student will also find that many general medical conditions produce changes in the eye. The eyeball consists of three tunics. The outer tunic is fibrous and composed of the sclera behind and the cornea in front. The middle tunic, or uveal tract, is a vascular coat composed of the choroid, the ciliary body, and the iris. The innermost tunic is the retina. Enclosed within the globe is the lens, with the aqueous humour in front and the vitreous body behind.

1. The fibrous tunic

The sclera is a dense fibrous membrane whose outer surface appears white. Internally it is separated from the choroid by a perichoroidal space. At the back of the eyeball the sclera is pierced by the optic nerve fibres at a region called the 'lamina cribrosa sclerae'. In the middle of the lamina the central artery and vein pierce the sclera. The ciliary nerves and vessels pierce the sclera around the optic nerve, and run forwards on the deep surface of the sclera. Further forwards the sclera is pierced by several venae vorticosae. In front, the sclera is continued as the cornea, the junction between the two being called the 'limbus'. An endothelial lined canal in the sclera runs around the periphery of the anterior chamber just behind the limbus (Fig. 3.22). It is the 'sinus venosus sclerae', or the 'canal of Schlemm'. The pectinate ligament of the iridocorneal angle separates the sinus venosus sclerae and the anterior chamber of the eye, and consists of a trabecular network of fibres extending between the posterior surface of the cornea and the base of the iris. Aqueous humour filters through these so-called 'spaces of Fontana' to the sinus and thence to the ciliary veins. A supporting ridge called the 'scleral spur' extends around the anterior chamber behind the sinus venosus sclerae. It gives attachment to ciliary muscle fibres and the ciliary body, and from here the iris can be traced radially into the aqueous humour. The iridocorneal angle is an important junction, and because of its relationship to the sinus venosus sclerae is often referred to as the 'filtration angle'. Abnormalities in this region may interfere with filtration of the aqueous humour and lead to an increase in intraocular pressure, a condition called 'glaucoma'.

The cornea is a non-vascular structure, the vessels of the sclera ending close to its circumference. The cornea therefore receives its nutrition by diffusion from the aqueous humour. There are no lymph vessels in the cornea. On the other hand,

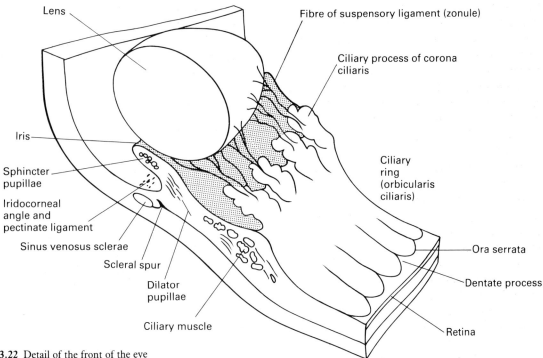

Lens

Fibre of suspensory ligament (zonule)

Ciliary process of corona ciliaris

Iris

Ciliary ring (orbicularis ciliaris)

Sphincter pupillae

Iridocorneal angle and pectinate ligament

Sinus venosus sclerae

Scleral spur

Dilator pupillae

Ciliary muscle

Ora serrata

Dentate process

Retina

Fig. 3.22 Detail of the front of the eye

it is highly sensitive, and many branches of the ophthalmic nerve are found around the periphery of the cornea where they form an annular plexus. From here they radiate into the cornea as a subepithelial plexus, where fine fibrils end between the epithelial cells as an intraepithelial plexus. Sensation from the cornea is carried through *both* the short and long ciliary nerves to the nasociliary nerve. The sensory fibres have their cell bodies in the trigeminal ganglion.

2. The vascular tunic or uveal tract

The vascular tunic consists of the choroid, the ciliary body and the iris. The choroid is highly vascular, and long and short posterior ciliary arteries reach it. Its outer surface is loosely connected to the sclera by the suprachoroid lamina, but the retina is firmly attached to its internal surface. Behind, the choroid is pierced by the optic nerve. The choroid is composed of three layers, the external layer being a vascular one, containing numerous small arteries and veins in a connective

tissue framework. The vascular layer contains branches of the posterior ciliary arteries which, after piercing the sclera around the optic nerve, stream forwards around the globe. They converge as vascular whorls where blood is collected into vorticose veins. There are four or five such veins, and these drain through the sclera into the ophthalmic veins. The intermediate layer of the choroid contains a very fine capillary network, which helps to nourish the outer layers of the retina. The innermost layer of the choroid is a fairly structureless membrane, called the 'membrane of Bruch.'

In front, the choroid can be traced to the ciliary body. This body is anchored to the scleral spur, and is attached to the lens by fine fibres. It is therefore concerned with suspension of the periphery of the lens and, because of the ciliary muscle it contains, is also capable of altering the pull on this suspension. The pull of the ciliary muscle *slackens the suspension* and allows the lens to adopt a highly convex form, and bulge towards the interior of the eyeball. The front of the ciliary body is related to the aqueous chamber of the eye, and is involved in the production of aqueous humour.

It is also possible that the ciliary body secretes mucopolysaccharides into the vitreous body. When viewed from the posterior chamber, the line of division between the choroid and ciliary body is scalloped. This edge is called the 'ora serrata'. Dentate processes of retina extend along the edges between the scallops, and may be traced onto the surface of the ciliary body. Here the retina is only two cell layers thick. It is, however, firmly attached, and if the choroid and retina separate, the retina tears at the ora serrata. Traced further forwards, the scallops give way to linear ridges. The section of the ciliary body made up of the scallops and ridges is called the 'ciliary ring' ('orbicularis ciliaris'). It is a relatively avascular region, and so incisions may be made in it for removal of intraocular foreign bodies. Traced further forwards, the ciliary body surface is deeply ridged by many ciliary processes, and this part of the body is called the 'corona ciliaris'. Suspensory ligament fibres of the lens are attached to the processes and to the grooves between them. The ciliary muscle fibres arise from the scleral spur and pass in several directions into the body. The most posterior fibres are long and pass in a meridional direction into the ciliary body where they terminate in star-like processes. Further forward are oblique fibres and a few sphincteric muscle fibres. The muscle of the ciliary body is supplied by postganglionic parasympathetic fibres from the ciliary ganglion. Contraction of the muscle slackens the pull on the suspensory ligament (zonule) of the lens, and allows it to bulge. Some sympathetic fibres also reach the ciliary body but these are probably concerned with blood vessel innervation.

At the iridocorneal angle, the ciliary body may be traced forwards as the iris, and adjustable diaphragm which surrounds the pupil. The iris contains pigment cells. If there is little pigment the iris appears blue, and if there are many melanocytes the iris is brown in colour. In the fetus the pupil is closed by a delicate pupillary membrane, but absorption of this begins at the sixth month of intrauterine life. The iris divides the aqueous chamber into two compartments, anterior and posterior. The ciliary processes protrude in the posterior of the chambers between the iris and the lens, and it is here that most of the aqueous fluid is produced. It circulates through the pupil into the anterior of the compartments and filters into the scleral venous sinus in the iridocorneal angle. The iris contains two sets of non-striated muscle fibres, the sphincter pupillae and the dilator pupillae. Postganglionic parasympathetic fibres from the short ciliary nerves innervate the sphincter pupillae. The dilator pupillae is supplied by postganglionic sympathetic fibres, which may reach the dilator either through the ciliary ganglion and short ciliary nerves or via the long ciliary nerves.

3. The retina

The retina is the sensory layer of the eyeball. Its internal surface is in contact with the hyaloid membrane of the vitreous body. It is continued outwards as the optic nerve at the back of the eyeball and ends at the ora serrata in front, where thin processes are continued onto the surface of the ciliary body. Near the centre of the posterior part of the retina is a small pale yellow area called the 'macula lutea'. This presents a central depression, the fovea centralis, where visual resolution is at its highest. The retina is thin at the fovea because some of the layers are absent. The optic nerve pierces the eyeball at the optic disc 3 mm to the nasal side of the macula. The circumference of the disc is raised, while the central part presents a shallow depression. The centre of the disc is pierced by the central artery and central vein of the retina. The optic disc is insensitive to light and is therefore sometimes called the 'blind spot'.

4. The aqueous humour, lens and vitreous body

The section of the eye in front of the lens is divided into anterior and posterior chambers by the iris. This part of the globe contains the aqueous humour, a fluid formed by active transport and diffusion from the capillaries of the ciliary processes in the angle between the lens and the iris. From here, aqueous humour circulates through the pupillary aperture into the anterior chamber. It escapes into the sinus venosus sclerae, and thence to the blood stream. Both lens and cornea are avascular and are nourished through the aqueous humour.

The vitreous body occupies the vitreous chamber of the eyeball. In front, it is hollowed into a concavity called the 'hyaloid fossa' into which the lens protrudes. At the periphery, the jelly-like vitreous body is limited by a hyaloid membrane. A narrow canal, the hyaloid canal, runs from the optic disc to the centre of the posterior surface of the lens. In the fetus this canal is occupied by the hyaloid artery, but this disappears a few weeks before birth. In front, the hyaloid membrane splits into two layers, one of which lines the hyaloid fossa, and the other forms a set of zonular fibres which are attached to the capsule of the lens.

The lens is a colourless structure covered with a capsule. It is described as having anterior and posterior poles, and a circumference called the 'equator'. A line connecting the anterior and posterior poles is the axis of the lens. In old age the lens becomes more flattened on both surfaces and slightly opaque. Severe opacity of the lens is called a 'cataract'. Very small opacities commonly occur in the aqueous humour and vitreous body. They move across the field of vision as the eye is moved, and are called 'floaters'. Although they sometimes cause concern to patients, they are usually not of serious significance.

CASE 4

Wanda Willow, a 14-year-old schoolgirl, was struck in the right eye with a stick during a hockey match. Initial examination was carried out in the accident unit. There was bruising of the eyelid and a small subconjunctival haemorrhage. Visual acuity, however, was normal. There was no evidence of perforation of the globe or injury to the iris. There was a small collection of blood at the base of the anterior chamber of the eye. The ophthalmoscope was then used to examine the eye more closely.

Wanda was asked to look straight ahead, and fix the eyes on a distant object. The light of the ophthalmoscope was directed into the eye, and the examining physician saw a 'red reflex'. Such a reflex indicated that the retina was not obscured by opacities in the cornea, lens or humour. With the ophthalmoscope set in the zero position, i.e. with no lens at the aperture of the instrument, the ophthalmoscope was moved close to Wanda's eye. The light was directed medially, and not straight into the eye. This direction allowed examination of the optic disc. (If the light is shone directly along the axis of the eye, it is directed on the macula, and the pupil constricts.) In order to see the disc clearly, adjustments were made to the ophthalmoscope head so that a lens strong enough to correct Wanda's refractive error was selected. (Plus lenses are used when the eye is long-sighted, and minus lenses when the eye is short-sighted.) The optic disc was normal, and appeared as a cup-shaped area paler than the surrounding fundus. The edge of this disc was sharp and well defined. The branches of the central artery were seen radiating over the edges of the disc. They were smaller and paler than the veins. At points where they crossed veins, the vein walls could be seen through the artery, and the calibre of the vein was normal. (Congestion of the optic disc, from raised intracranial pressure, is called 'papilloedema' — the optic cup is obscured and the disc margin blurred.) The macula was finally inspected and was normal. Wanda therefore had a fairly normal eye, apart from a small collection of blood in the anterior chamber. This collection cleared slowly during the subsequent weeks.

Provided that there is no contraindication, the pupil may be dilated by using a mydriatic; this makes inspection of the fundus easier. It is especially useful when examining the macula, because pupillary constriction does not occur. A greater area of retina can also be examined by this method.

Binocular colour vision is an asset which man shares with only a few other groups of animals. It is therefore precious. Many conditions affect the eye and its function, and include both local disease and general problems such as hypertension and diabetes. Patients with ocular problems will frequently need to be seen by an ophthalmologist, but the student should be able to conduct an initial examination of the eye and its surrounding structures. Such an examination must always include an assessment of visual acuity, tests for eye movements and ophthalmoscopy.

4

THE PETROUS TEMPORAL BONE AND THE EAR

THE TEMPORAL BONE

A preliminary study of some of the features of the temporal bone will reward the student with a better understanding of the ear and its relationships to neurovascular structures. These latter structures include the 7th, 8th, 9th and 10th cranial nerves, the internal carotid artery with its sympathetic plexus, and the internal jugular vein.

The temporal bone consists of four morphological sections — the petrous and squamous parts, the tympanic plate, and the styloid process. The simplest way to build up a picture of the bone and the relationships of these constituents to each other is to examine the fetal state. The air-containing part of the ear develops as a diverticulum of the primitive pharynx called the 'tubotympanic recess' (Fig. 4.1A). The end of this tube reaches the surface where it will form the tympanic membrane. The dorsal ends of the first two branchial cartilages are also closely related to the recess. Most of the first arch cartilage, Meckel's cartilage, degenerates, but part of the cartilage associated with the recess remains trapped in the developing temporal bone and contributes to the development of the malleus and incus of the middle ear. The dorsal part of the second arch cartilage gives rise to the stapes of the middle ear and to the styloid process. The muscle of the stapes, the stapedius, is developed from second arch mesoderm and is supplied by the second arch nerve, the facial nerve, a cranial nerve closely related to the developing ear. The organs of hearing and balance develop within a mass of mesenchyme which soon chondrifies. Ossification takes place in this cartilage to make the petrous part of

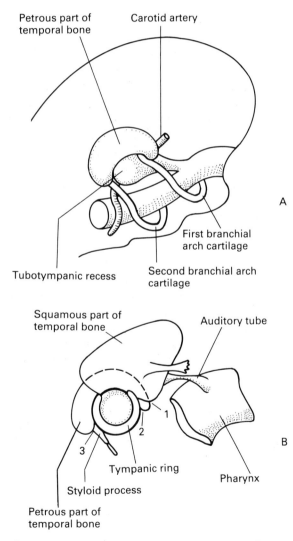

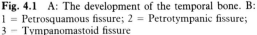

Fig. 4.1 A: The development of the temporal bone. B: 1 = Petrosquamous fissure; 2 = Petrotympanic fissure; 3 = Tympanomastoid fissure

the temporal bone. The bone forms close to the future internal carotid artery, and this becomes enveloped, so that it comes to lie in a carotid canal. The posterior part of the petrous temporal bone contains a small extension from the tubo-tympanic recess called the 'mastoid antrum'. This air cavity is well-formed at birth. The mastoid process, however, is not formed at birth. Where the tubotympanic recess is in contact with the surface, a tympanic ring of bone develops by ossification in membrane (Fig. 4.1B). The ring is open above. In the fetal skull, the tympanic membrane is close to the surface, and it is only later that the ring develops into a broader and longer tympanic plate. The squamous part of the temporal bone develops separately and ossifies in membrane. The petrous part of the temporal bone is thus found *behind, above and wedged in front* of the tubotympanic recess. This part of the recess develops into the middle ear cavity. The narrow section of the recess which joins the pharynx in front will become the auditory tube. The petrous bone which forms the roof of the middle ear is thin, and called the 'tegmen tympani'. The lower edge of the tegmen is wedged between the squamous part of the temporal bone and the tympanic plate. In this way several fissures may be identified. In front of the external acoustic meatus is the squamotympanic fissure. This, traced downwards to the base of the skull, is divided by the edge of the tegmen tympani (petrous bone) into the petro-squamous and petrotympanic fissures. At the back of the external acoustic meatus is a tympano-mastoid fissure. The suture between the petrous and squamous parts of the temporal bone remains unossified during the first few years of life, and ear infections may pass directly into the cranial cavity by this route. Although the suture ossifies, veins traverse it between the ear and the superior petrosal sinus. Thus there remains in the adult a means of spreading infection from the ear to the cranial cavity.

THE EAR

The ear may be divided into three parts — the external ear, the middle ear and the internal ear.

1. The external ear

The outer ear consists of the auricle and the external acoustic meatus. The skeleton of the auricle is made of elastic fibrocartilage. The surface is irregular and composed of numerous depressions and eminences. Its sensory nerve supply is described in Chapter 12. Both the external acoustic meatus and the tympanic membrane may be examined with the aid of an otoscope. In the newborn child the meatus is short, and great care should therefore be exercised when conducting such an examination. The meatus elongates as the tympanic ring becomes transformed into a tympanic plate. The outer third of the meatus is cartilaginous, and only the inner section is walled by bone. Most of the bone is formed by the tympanic plate, but a small amount of the roof is formed by the squamous part of the temporal bone. During the first few years of life, a hole called the 'foramen of Huschke' is found in the anterior wall of the osseous part of the external acoustic meatus. It is filled with connective tissue, but this usually ossifies during childhood.

The meatus is not straight, but forms an S-shaped curve. Traced inwards, it first curves anteriorly and then posteriorly, finally veering antero-inferiorly to reach the tympanic membrane. This membrane is not set at right angles to the meatus but is placed obliquely so that the anterior wall and floor of the meatus are longer than the roof and posterior wall. In order to straighten the meatus for otoscopic examination the auricle should be pulled upwards and backwards. There are two constrictions in the meatus, the narrowest of which occurs at the junction of the cartilaginous and bony parts of the tube. There is a further constriction, the isthmus, in the osseous part of the meatus close to the tympanic membrane. A foreign body, accidentally inserted into the meatus by a child, may become impacted at one of the constricted parts of the meatus. Numerous ceruminous glands are found in the subcutaneous tissue of the cartilaginous part of the meatus, and these secrete 'wax' or 'cerumen'. Protective meatal hairs also occur near the opening of the meatus. Rarely, developmental abnormalities such as pre-auricular cysts and sinuses may be found close to the auricle.

There is a fibrocartilaginous ring around the periphery of the tympanic membrane which is attached to the tympanic sulcus in the bone of the meatus. The appearance of the normal membrane during otoscopic examination is characteristic (Fig. 4.2). Certain parts of the malleus shine through the membrane. The long handle of the bone is attached to the inner surface of the membrane and can be seen as a streak passing downwards and backwards to a point just below its centre. At the upper end of the handle a small lateral process of the bone makes a prominence on the membrane. Anterior and posterior folds extend upwards from this to the periphery of the membrane. Enclosed between the folds is a flaccid part of the membrane, which is particularly vascular and which has the chorda tympani on its deep surface. The handle of the malleus draws the tympanic membrane inwards so that the outer surface of the membrane is concave. The light from the otoscope produces a cone of reflected light in the anteroinferior quadrant of the membrane.

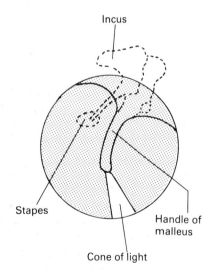

Fig. 4.2 The tympanic membrane

2. The middle ear

a. The middle ear structure and the ossicles

The middle ear or tympanic cavity is a small space lined with mucoperiosteum and filled with air. It communicates with the pharynx in front through the auditory tube, and with the mastoid antrum behind by means of an aditus. The upper part of the cavity is expanded into an epitympanic recess. The middle ear contains a chain of three ossicles connecting the tympanic membrane to the medial wall of the middle ear, and these transmit vibrations across the cavity from the external to the internal ear. There is thus an intricate mechanical coupling between the vibrations of the tympanic membrane and vibrations of the fluid in the inner ear.

Although the tympanic cavity is in reality irregular in shape, it is best described as having lateral, medial, anterior and posterior walls, a roof and a floor (Fig. 4.3). The lateral wall is formed by the tympanic membrane. The medial wall is the bone of the inner ear, and presents several eminences and grooves produced by inner ear structures. The promontory is a rounded elevation produced by the underlying cochlea. Just behind this are two openings in the bone which lead into the bony labyrinth of the inner ear. The upper opening is the fenestra vestibuli, and is closed in life by the footplate of the stapes. This bone is attached to the edge of the opening by an annular ligament. The lower opening is the fenestra cochleae, and is closed with a secondary tympanic membrane, which like the tympanic membrane proper, has a concave outer surface. A bulge near the upper part of the medial wall of the middle ear indicates the position of a canal conducting the facial nerve. Behind this is an eminence produced by the lateral semicircular canal. The anterior wall of the tympanic cavity leads to two canals — the auditory tube and the canal for the tensor tympani muscle. The auditory tube is the lower and larger of the two, and slopes at 30° to the horizontal, as it passes medially towards the pharynx. The canal is at first within the petrous part of the temporal bone, but is continued to the pharynx as a cartilaginous tube. This cartilaginous section occupies the groove between the petrous temporal bone and the greater wing of the sphenoid on the undersurface of the skull, and opens into the nasopharynx. The narrowest part of the auditory tube is found at the junction between the bony and cartilaginous parts. The tube acts as a protective mechanism for the middle ear allowing pressure to be equalised

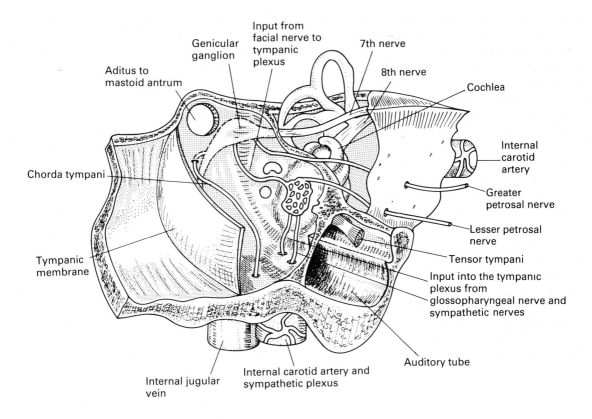

Fig. 4.3 The middle ear

on the two sides of the tympanic membrane at all times. The tube is opened during deglutition and the cartilaginous part is related to several muscles which could assist in this process. The tensor veli palatini, levator veli palatini and the salpingopharyngeus muscles are close to and partly arise from the tube (see Ch. 11). Some fibres of the tensor palati are said to attach to the cartilage of the tube and are known as the 'dilatator tubae', but all three of these muscles probably assist in opening the tube during deglutition. Above the auditory tube is a canal for the tensor tympani muscle. This small muscle enters the tympanic cavity and gives rise to a delicate tendon which changes direction to reach its insertion into the handle of the malleus. It does this by passing around a small bony pulley called the 'processus trochleariformis'. The carotid canal is related to the anterior wall of the middle ear, with only a thin lamina of bone separating the two.

The posterior wall of the tympanic cavity is in-timately associated with the mastoid antrum. An opening, the aditus, leads from the epitympanic recess into the mastoid antrum. A small pyramidal eminence containing the stapedius muscle is found on the posterior wall below the aditus. The tendon of this muscle emerges through the summit of the pyramid, and travels from here to its insertion into the stapes. The roof of the tympanic cavity is thin and formed by part of the petrous temporal bone called the 'tegmen tympani'. Above it are the meninges and the temporal lobe of the brain. The floor of the tympanic cavity is narrow and related to the jugular foramen, the superior bulb of the internal jugular vein, the glossopharyngeal nerve, the vagus nerve, and the accessory nerve.

The tympanic cavity contains three ossicles — the malleus, incus and stapes. These are united by synovial joints, a saddle-shaped articulation between malleus and incus and a ball-and-socket articulation between the incus and stapes. The malleus is said to look like a hammer, its head lying in the epitympanic recess. It is held in place by superior and lateral ligaments. The neck is the constricted part of the bone below the head, and bears a pointed anterior process from which an anterior ligament extends to the wall of the tympanic cavity. This ligament is connected through the petrotympanic fissure in the fetus to Meckel's cartilage. Indeed, the malleus and incus represent the trapped dorsal end of the cartilage. The handle of the malleus is firmly attached to the inner surface of the tympanic membrane. It articulates posteriorly with the incus. The incus has a body and long and short processes. A ligament attaches the short process to the bone of the epitympanic recess. At the end of the long process is a rounded projection which forms the 'ball' of the joint between the incus and stapes. The stapes resembles a stirrup in shape. In its head is a concavity which is the 'socket' for the synovial articulation between it and the incus. Two limbs extend from the head to the footplate, which is attached to the margin of the fenestra vestibuli by an annular ligament. The stapes represents the trapped dorsal end of the second arch cartilage of the embryo.

Vibrations from the tympanic membrane are transmitted to the footplate of the stapes which in turn rocks in the fenestra vestibuli. Its movements are complex, but any inward movement communicated to the perilymph is reflected in an outward bulging of the secondary tympanic membrane in the fenestra cochleae. The two muscles, the stapedius and tensor tympani, protect against excessive vibration in the ossicle chain. The tensor tympani attaches to the handle of the malleus close to its root, and the stapedius to the neck of the stapes. The nerve supply to tensor tympani arises below the petrous temporal bone in the infratemporal fossa. Here, a branch of the mandibular nerve (the nerve to the medial pterygoid) gives a small twig which enters the canal for the tensor tympani, and supplies the muscle. The mandibular nerve is the nerve of the first arch. The stapedius is supplied by the 7th cranial nerve, the nerve of the second arch.

CASE 1

Mangla Mould, a 45-year-old grocer's assistant,

had noticed progressive loss of hearing in the right ear over a period of 15 years. She also complained of ringing in the ear (tinnitus), and attacks of giddiness (vertigo). Both her parents had been hard of hearing, and Mangla believed that her deafness was familial. During recent months, however, she had noticed weakness and stiffness of the right side of the face and had three attacks of severe facial pain. She also suffered frequent occipital headaches. These latter symptoms eventually led her to a consultation at the neurosurgical clinic.

Examination showed marked right-sided deafness, weakness of the right facial muscles, a delayed right blinking reflex, and loss of sensation of the right cornea. Audiology and vestibulometry confirmed severe affliction of both cochlear and vestibular parts of the right vestibulocochlear nerve. A CT scan showed a large mass at the back of the right petrous temporal bone (Fig. 4.4). This was thought to be a tumour of the 8th cranial nerve, an acoustic neuroma. Such tumours usually grow from the nerve in the internal acoustic meatus, and cause pressure on the cochlear, vestibular and facial nerves. As the tumour enlarges it extends into the cerebellopontine angle. Here, it indents the brain stem, and is often closely related to the anterior inferior cerebellar artery. A large tumour may also involve other cranial nerves, and the depressed right corneal reflex found during examination of Mangla was an indication of pressure on the sensory part of the trigeminal nerve. Occasionally, a large tumour will compress the brain stem, and produce increase in the pressure of CSF within the brain (obstructive hydrocephalus).

Operation notes

Mangla was prepared for a posterior fossa craniotomy. After shaving the head, Mangla was anaesthetised and placed on her left side on the operating table. A lateral approach to the posterior cranial fossa was made through a hockey-stick incision. The vertical midline incision was started at the superior nuchal line, and curled towards the mastoid process at the lower end. The bone of the posterior cranial fossa was exposed by detaching overlying musculature. A burr hole was made, and the opening enlarged by nibbling away the bone edges. Bone removal extended from the transverse and sigmoid sinuses above to the foramen magnum below. It was taken as far laterally as the mastoid air cells. The cerebellum was retracted, and the large tumour exposed (Fig. 4.5). Removal was difficult, but complete. Following recovery, Mangla was left with a complete right-sided facial palsy. A few months later, however, at a further surgical procedure, the peripheral part of the facial nerve was joined to a cut hypoglossal nerve (facio-hypoglossal anastomosis). Although cutting the

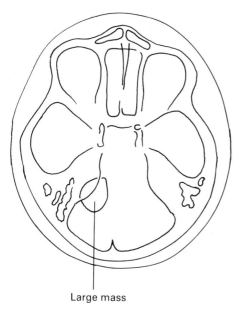

Large mass

A

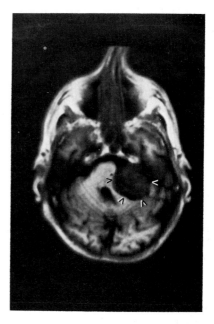

C

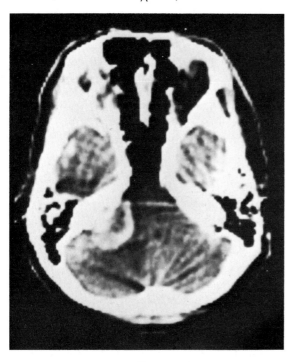

B

Fig. 4.4 Mangla Mould. A: Tracing of CT scan. B: CT scan
of head. (By kind permission of Mr L. Flood FRCS and Dr P.
Hamlyn, Royal Ear Hospital.) C: MRI scan. Inversion
recovery image showing a large acoustic neuroma (dark area
indicated by arrows). (By kind permission of Dr Jackie
Pennock and the NMR Unit of The Royal Postgraduate
Medical School, Hammersmith Hospital.)

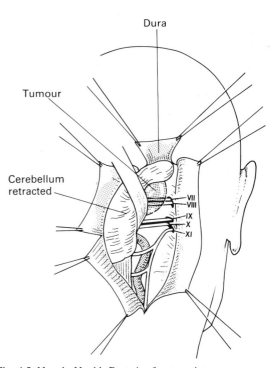

Dura

Tumour

Cerebellum
retracted

VII
VIII
IX
X
XI

Fig. 4.5 Mangla Mould. Posterior fossa craniotomy.

hypoglossal nerve in this way denervates the muscles of the side of the tongue, little disability is noticed. Mangla eventually regained tone in the right facial muscles, and was able to perform simple facial movements.

The tumour in this case was revealed by means of computed tomography, but an MRI scan would also have given this information. Figure 4.4C is a magnetic resonance imaging scan of another patient, and shows a large tumour in the cerebello-pontine angle. It has been surrounded by four arrows. The tumour, an acoustic neuroma, extends backwards from the petrous temporal bone into the cerebellum.

b. Nerve relations of the middle ear

Both facial and vestibulocochlear nerves enter the petrous temporal bone from the posterior cranial fossa through the internal acoustic meatus. The vestibulocochlear nerve divides at the lateral end of the internal acoustic meatus into cochlear and vestibular portions. The termination of this nerve is described in the section dealing with the internal ear. As the 7th and 8th cranial nerves approach the meatus, a bundle called the 'nervus intermedius' is attached to the vestibulocochlear nerve. At the meatus the 7th nerve lies in a groove on the upper surface of the vestibulocochlear nerve with the nervus intermedius between them. From here, the nervus intermedius is closely associated with the facial nerve, and is described as being part of it. The bone at the bottom of the meatus is divided into upper and lower areas by a transverse crest, and the facial nerve enters a bony canal above the crest. The nerve passes laterally in the canal above the vestibule to reach the medial wall of the epitympanic recess. It then turns sharply backwards towards the posterior wall of the tympanic cavity. The point where it bends is called the 'geniculum' and here the nerve presents an enlargement, the genicular ganglion. When it reaches the posterior wall of the tympanic cavity, the nerve lies close by the aditus to the mastoid antrum. Here it takes another bend, this time downwards, which takes it past the posterior wall of the tympanic cavity to leave the skull at the stylomastoid foramen. Parts of the wall of the facial nerve canal may be defficient.

During its intrapetrous course, the 7th nerve gives important branches, some of which communicate with neighbouring cranial nerves (Fig. 4.6). The greater petrosal nerve arises from the region of the genicular ganglion, and it belongs to the nervus intermedius. It is a mixed nerve sending preganglionic parasympathetic fibres to the pterygopalatine ganglion and conveying taste fibres from the palate. The greater petrosal nerve leaves the petrous temporal bone in the middle cranial fossa through a slit on its anterior slope. It runs deep to the trigeminal ganglion and Meckel's cave to reach the foramen lacerum, where it is joined by sympathetic fibres from the plexus around the internal carotid artery. The mixed bundle of parasympathetic and sympathetic fibres is called the 'nerve of the pterygoid canal'. The canal is found in the sphenoid bone below the foramen rotundum, at the root of the pterygoid plates. It transmits the mixture of fibres to the pterygopalatine ganglion. Here parasympathetic fibres synapse and are distributed along the branches of the ganglion to the glands of paranasal air sinuses, nose and nasopharynx. In addition there are fibres which join the zygomatic branch of the maxillary nerve. This takes them to the lateral wall of the orbit where they ascend in a communicating nerve to the lacrimal nerve. They hitch-hike along this nerve for a short distance to reach the lacrimal gland (see Ch. 3). The few taste fibres in the greater petrosal nerve have their cell bodies in the genicular ganglion of the facial nerve.

The facial nerve, while in the petrous temporal bone, sends a branch to the tympanic plexus, a plexus of nerves lying on the promontory of the medial wall of the tympanic cavity. The 7th nerve also sends a small twig through a canal in the bone to supply the stapedius muscle. Near the epitympanic recess, the chorda tympani leaves the facial nerve, crosses the tympanic cavity medial to the malleus, and leaves the skull through the petro-tympanic fissure (Fig. 4.7). It then grooves the medial side of the spine of the sphenoid and reaches the infratemporal fossa. Here, it joins the lingual nerve which carries its fibres to the floor of the mouth. The chorda tympani, like the greater petrosal branch, is a mixed nerve belonging to the nervus intermedius. It transmits taste fibres from the anterior two-thirds of the tongue

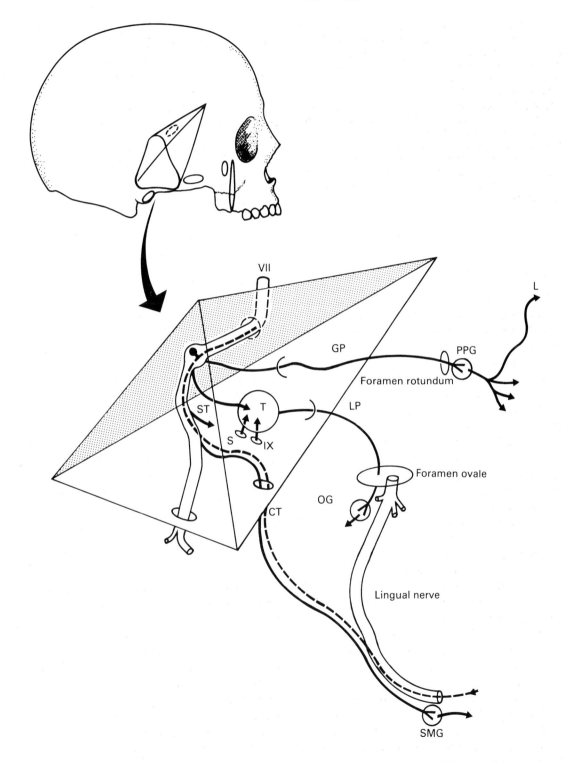

Fig. 4.6 The facial nerve. ST = nerve to stapedius; T = tympanic plexus; S = sympathetic fibres; CT = chorda tympani; OG = otic ganglion; SMG = submandibular ganglion; PPG = pterygopalatine ganglion; GP = greater petrosal nerve; LP = lesser petrosal nerve; L = nerve to lacrimal gland.

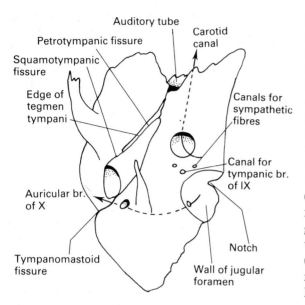

Fig. 4.7 The under surface of the temporal bone

and these have their cell bodies in the genicular ganglion. It also transmits preganglionic parasympathetic fibres which synapse in the floor of the mouth in the submandibular ganglion. Postganglionic fibres leave this ganglion for the submandibular, sublingual and mucous glands in the floor of the mouth (see Ch. 11).

Both glossopharyngeal and vagus nerves send fibres to the ear. The 9th cranial nerve leaves the posterior cranial fossa through a pyramidal notch in the petrous temporal bone on the edge of the jugular foramen. Once in this notch, the nerve gives a tympanic branch, sometimes called 'Jacobson's nerve'. It enters a small bony canal on the edge of the jugular foramen, and is transmitted to the middle ear and the tympanic plexus. The nerve contains sensory fibres responsible for sensation in the middle ear and the inner surface of the tympanic membrane. It also contains preganglionic parasympathetic fibres. These pass through the plexus and emerge in the form of the lesser petrosal nerve (Fig. 4.6). This leaves the petrous temporal bone through a slit on its anterior slope, and approaches the foramen ovale. It leaves the skull through this foramen and, in the infratemporal fossa, its parasympathetic fibres synapse in the otic ganglion. Postganglionic fibres hitch-hike

for a short distance along the auriculotemporal nerve to reach the parotid gland. A small branch of communication is usually found between the 7th cranial nerve and the lesser petrosal so that the fibres reaching the parotid are probably a mixture of 9th and 7th cranial nerve fibres. The tympanic plexus also has a small input from the 7th nerve, and from sympathetic fibres of the plexus around the internal carotid artery. These latter fibres ascend through small bony canals in the petrous temporal bone to reach the tympanic cavity (Fig. 4.7). As the vagus nerve enters the jugular foramen, it bears a swelling called the 'superior ganglion'. A small meningeal branch arises from this ganglion together with an auricular branch (sometimes called 'Arnold's nerve'). This latter nerve ascends through a small bony canal which leads to the tympanomastoid suture. Here it enters the external acoustic meatus and supplies sensory fibres to a small area of the upper part of the outer surface of the tympanic membrane. (The rest of the outer surface is supplied by the auriculotemporal branch of the mandibular nerve.) The auricular branch of the vagus also supplies a little skin in the meatus and a small area of skin in the groove at the back of the auricle.

It is obvious from the above account that several nerves and their branches are intimately related within the petrous part of the temporal bone, and communicating branches often occur between these nerves. One such communication occurs between the 7th nerve and the auricular branch of the vagus. The Ramsay Hunt syndrome is a herpes infection of the genicular ganglion and gives rise to vesicles on the outer surface of the tympanic membrane. These 7th nerve fibres are probably carried there via the communicating branch of the facial nerve to the auricular branch of the vagus.

CASE 2

Humphrey Limpit, a 35-year-old deep-sea fisherman, had suffered from recurrent infections in the right ear since childhood. Several of these infections had been severe, and accompanied by discharge from the ear. He had been told that the right ear drum had perforated during one of these infections. Humphrey wore a cotton wool plug in the ear when he went fishing in order to prevent

THE PETROUS TEMPORAL BONE AND THE EAR 71

sea water entering the meatus. Recently, he had noticed a 'stiffness' of the muscles of the right side of the face, but thought that this was a 'chill'. He consulted his physician because of a recurrent attack of severe ear pain.

On examination he was found to have no discharge from the ear, but had a large old central perforation on the drum. He had weakness of the facial muscles on the right side of the face. Taste was tested on the anterior two-thirds of the tongue. There was lack of sensation to taste on the right side. A Schirmer's test was then conducted to assess lacrimal secretion. A small strip of blotting paper was placed into the lower conjunctival fornix of each eye, and left in place for five minutes. When the two pieces of blotting paper were compared, there was a marked decrease in lacrimation on the right. Audiology showed that the cochlear nerve was also affected, but no abnormality of the vestibular nerve was detected. The clinical signs indicated that the lesion was mainly affecting the facial nerve, and its chorda tympani and greater petrosal branches. This was confirmed with CT, which showed a lucent area with clearly

outlined bony margins expanding the facial canal (Figs. 4.8, 4.9). This was thought to be a cholesteatoma. This chronic growth grows slowly in the ear and mastoid, and erodes adjacent structures. The growth was removed by exposing the facial canal with the aid of a dissecting microscope. At operation, the stretched facial nerve was preserved, and Humphrey made a good recovery.

c. The mastoid antrum and mastoid process

The mastoid antrum, an air sinus within the petrous part of the temporal bone, lies behind the middle ear. Unlike the other air sinuses it is well developed at birth, although the mastoid process itself is not formed at this time. The mastoid antrum is important clinically because of the possibility of spread of infection into it from the middle ear. It is also sometimes used as a surgical route to the middle ear. Its position may be mapped on the surface of the skull just above and behind the

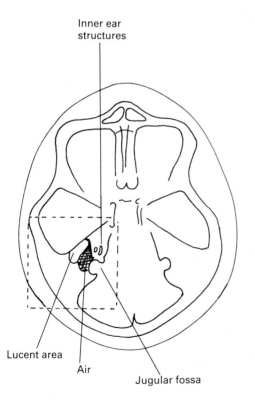

Inner ear structures

Lucent area

Air

Jugular fossa

A

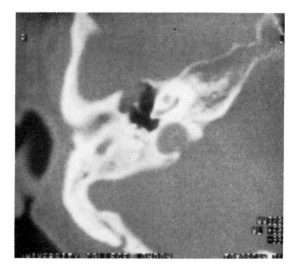

B

Fig. 4.8 Humphrey Limpit. A: Tracing of CT scan. B: CT scan of head

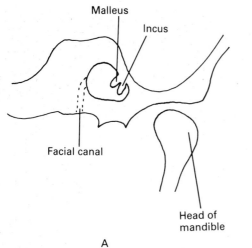

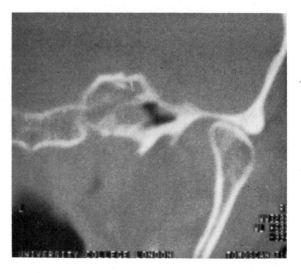

A   B

Fig. 4.9 A: Tracing from CT scan of the petrous temporal bone (longitudinal sections). The malleus and incus together give the so-called 'molar tooth' appearance. B: CT scan of the petrous temporal bone (longitudinal sections).

external acoustic meatus. Here, there is a depression called the 'suprameatal triangle'. Above, the triangle is formed by the supramastoid crest. The anterior boundary is formed by the superior margin of the external acoustic meatus, and is also the surface mark for the descending part of the facial nerve. A vertical line forms the posterior margin and completes the triangle. The aditus in the anterior wall of the mastoid antrum leads from the epitympanic recess. Posteriorly, the mastoid antrum is related to the sigmoid sinus, and here the bone may be quite thin. An emissary vein frequently passes from the sigmoid sinus through a bony canal in the base of the mastoid process to veins of the occiput. The roof of the antrum, like that of the tympanic cavity, is formed by the tegmen tympani. The antrum is related to the meninges and the brain through the roof. The medial wall of the antrum is related to the posterior semicircular canal and in front to the descending part of the facial nerve.

The mastoid process itself does not begin to develop until the second year of life, and then air cells gradually extend into it. The extent to which the mastoid process is pneumatised, however, is variable (Fig. 4.10). Some mastoids are well developed while others have few or no air cells. The air cavities are lined with mucoperiosteum and are continuous with the air-containing mastoid antrum

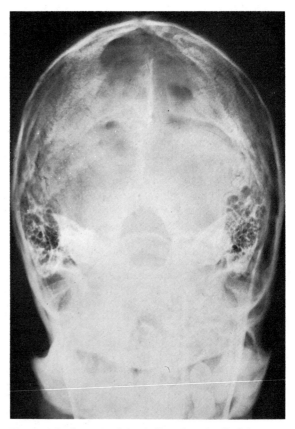

Fig. 4.10 Radiograph of the skull to show detail of the mastoid processes

and the tympanic cavity. Occasionally, air cells are found in other parts of the petrous temporal bone. A group of air cells often extends to the apex of the petrous temporal bone. These apical air cells are related to the auditory tube, the carotid canal, and to the labyrinth. Two nerves also lie close to the apex of the temporal bone; the abducent nerve often grooves the bone as it pierces the inferior petrosal sinus, and the trigeminal ganglion lies on the upper surface of the apex in Meckel's cave. Infection in this apical group of air cells can extend to all these related structures. The sensory nerve supply to the mastoid antrum and air cells comes from the meningeal branch of the mandibular nerve (nervus spinosus).

CASE 3

Ulrich Koch, a 40-year-old market gardener, developed severe pain in both ears after an attack of influenza. She put drops into the ears over several days, but eventually consulted her doctor because there was no improvement. When she was seen she had a small perforation in the left ear drum and discharge was seeping through the hole from the middle ear. The right drum was red and inflamed. She was given a course of antibiotics. The discharge continued, and the pain did not improve. Ulrich also noticed that she saw 'double' when looking to the left, and on examination she was found to have weakness of the left lateral rectus muscle. She was referred for a specialist opinion. The clue to her condition came from a submentovertical radiograph of the base of the skull (Fig. 4.11). The apices of both petrous temporal bones showed a fuzzy obliteration of detail, and the foramina were unclear. This was because there was osteomyelitis of the apices of the petrous temporal bones. Compare the picture with that of Figure 1.18 in Chapter 1, which is a normal radiograph of the skull base. Note the position of the apex of the petrous temporal bone, and the foramen spinosum and foramen ovale in the sphenoid. Ulrich had infection of the air cells at the apices of the petrous temporal bones, and the infection had affected the 6th left cranial nerve. Such infections, while not common, can affect any of the structures around the apex of the petrous temporal bone. These include the 6th cranial nerve, the internal carotid artery and its sympathetic plexus, the greater petrosal nerve, and the trigeminal ganglion. Ulrich was admitted to hospital and treated with intravenous antibiotics. The condition was halted, but she was left with permanent weakness of the left lateral rectus.

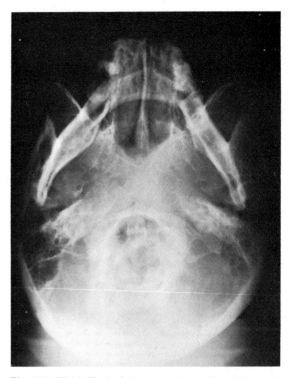

Fig. 4.11 Ulrich Koch. Submentovertical radiograph.

Infections in any part of the petrous temporal bone can spread to adjacent structures. Middle ear infection (otitis media) can spread to the mastoid process and produce a mastoiditis. It can spread upwards through the tegmen tympani to the meninges and temporal lobe of the brain, even producing a temporal lobe abscess. Spread into the sigmoid sinus can lead to thrombosis. Infections of the petrous temporal bone, therefore, whether in the middle ear, mastoid or petrous apex, must be carefully monitored during treatment.

3. The inner ear

The petrous temporal bone is excavated to form a series of cavities and canals called the 'bony labyrinth'. The organs of hearing and balance fit inside this complex network as the membranous labyrinth.

a. The bony labyrinth

The bony labyrinth consists of a centrally placed cavern called the 'vestibule' which communicates behind with three semicircular canals, and in front leads to a curled canal, the cochlea (Fig. 4.12). The bony labyrinth contains perilymph whose composition closely resembles that of cerebrospinal fluid. Indeed, there is an aqueduct which passes through the petrous temporal bone from the base of the cochlea to the pyramidal notch in the jugular foramen (Fig. 4.13). Here it is continuous with the subarachnoid space. It is said that there is a slow continuous flow of cerebrospinal fluid along this aqueduct. It is likely, however, that perilymph also originates as a transudate from blood vessels in the walls of the bony labyrinth. Perilymph is probably removed through the aqueduct of the cochlea, but other methods of removal cannot be excluded.

The fenestra vestibuli is an opening on the lateral wall of the vestibule, and is closed in life by the footplate of the stapes. Movement of the stapes therefore sets up vibrations in the perilymph of the vestibule. The posterior vestibular wall is perfor-

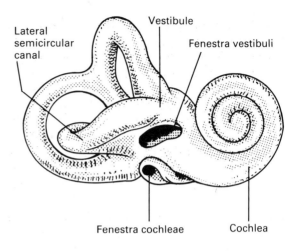

Fig. 4.12 The bony labyrinth

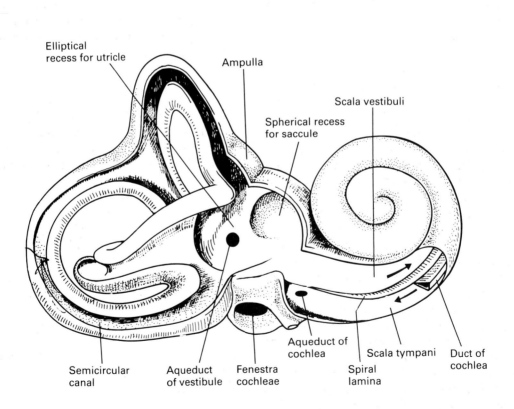

Fig. 4.13 The interior of the bony labyrinth

ated by numerous holes for the passage of the fibres of the vestibular part of the vestibulocochlear nerve. These enter the inner ear from the fundus of the internal acoustic meatus, which lies on the medial side of this wall. In the centre of the posterior wall, the aqueduct of the vestibule leads to an opening on the posterior slope of the petrous temporal bone. It does not transmit perilymph because it is completely filled by the membranous ductus endolymphaticus. The cochlea is a sinuous tunnel which runs forwards from the cavity of the vestibule. It resembles the shell of a snail, with about two and three-quarter turns. The apex of the cochlea, the cupula, lies deep to the medial wall of the tympanic cavity, where it raises a bulge called the 'promontory'. The cochlea is wound around a central axis called the 'modiolus'. Its canal is partially divided by an osseous spiral lamina, which projects from the central column into the canal. The division of the canal of the cochlea is completed by a basilar membrane which stretches from the edge of the spiral lamina to a spiral ligament on the outer wall of the canal. The canal of the cochlea is thus completely divided into a scala vestibuli above and a scala tympani below (Figs. 4.13, 4.15). The two canals are continuous through a gap at the apex of the cochlea called the 'helicotrema'. Vibrations in the perilymph, created by movement of the footplate of the stapes, travel along the curved scala vestibuli to the apex of the cochlea. Here they pass through the helicotrema into the scala tympani, and travel downwards to the base of the cochlea. This leads to the fenestra cochleae, which is closed in life by the secondary tympanic membrane. Movements occur in this membrane in the opposite direction to those of the footplate of the stapes, so that pressure in the inner ear perilymph does not become excessive. The base of the cochlea lies against the bottom of the internal acoustic meatus, and is pierced by numerous foramina which transmit fibres of the cochlear part of the vestibulocochlear nerve. The foramina have a spiral orientation, reflecting the spiral arrangement of the cochlea, and the perforated substance is called the 'tractus spiralis foraminosus'. From here, fibres pass to bony canals in the modiolus and thence in canals which carry them to the base of the osseous spiral lamina. The canals along the margin of the lamina are enlarged

as a spiral canal, and this lodges the spiral ganglion of the nerve.

Semicircular canals lead posteriorly from the vestibule, and are named 'anterior' ('superior'), 'posterior', and 'lateral'. At one end, each presents a dilatation called an 'ampulla'. The anterior (superior) and posterior canals are vertically placed, the posterior canal lying in the long axis of the petrous temporal bone and the anterior canal lying at right angles to this axis. The anterior canal lies at a higher level than the posterior canal when the head is held in the horizontal position, and this is why it is often called the 'superior' canal. It produces the arcuate eminence on the petrous temporal bone. One limb of the anterior canal joins a limb of the posterior canal to form a common opening. At the points where the ampullae of the canals join the vestibule there are small holes which conduct fibres of the vestibular part of the 8th cranial nerve. The bundle of fibres to the posterior semicircular canal ampulla is separate from the others and leaves the bottom of the internal acoustic meatus through the foramen singulare. The lateral semicircular canal lies horizontally, and its convexity gives rise to a bulge in the medial wall of the tympanic cavity.

b. The membranous labyrinth

The cavities and canals of the bony labyrinth contain a series of membranous sacs and tubes filled with endolymph (Fig. 4.14). This membranous labyrinth is smaller than the cavities and canals of

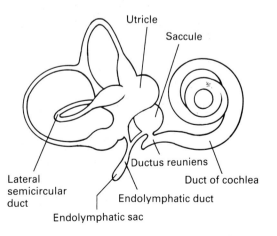

Fig. 4.14 The membranous labyrinth

the bony labyrinth. Two sacs of endolymph lie within the vestibule — the utricle behind and the saccule in front. The utricle is the larger of the sacs and produces an elliptical recess on the posterior wall of the vestibule (Fig. 4.13). The saccule makes a smaller spherical recess on the posterior wall of the vestibule. Semicircular ducts are continuous posteriorly with the utricle and lie within the semicircular canals. In front, the cochlear duct lies within the cochlea.

A tiny canal, the ductus utriculosaccularis, leads to the ductus endolymphaticus. This structure with its dilated end, the saccus endolymphaticus, occupies the aqueduct of the vestibule. The saccus lies beneath the dura on the posterior slope of the petrous temporal bone where it is covered by a cap of specialised epithelial cells and a vascular plexus. It is likely that these latter structures are responsible for removal of endolymph. The saccule is joined to the duct of the cochlea in front by the ductus reuniens. Both utricle and saccule contain specialised neuroepithelium. Part of the floor and lateral wall of the utricle is thickened by a specialised organ called the 'macula'. A similar thickening is found in the anterior wall of the saccule — the macula of the saccule, which is set at right angles to the macula of the utricle. Three semicircular ducts occupy the semicircular canals of the bony labyrinth. They open by means of five orifices into the utricle, an anterior and posterior duct sharing one orifice. Near the orifices the ducts are dilated as ampullae, and each contains a projection called an 'ampullary crest'.

The maculae of the utricle and saccule signal alterations in the position of the head with reference to the pull of gravity. Much of the information from these organs produces appropriate alterations in muscle tone throughout the body. The supporting muscles, muscles of the neck and muscles concerned with eye movements are particularly affected. The maculae are therefore sometimes referred to as the 'organs of static balance', but they possibly have other functions. The ampullary crests of the semicircular canals, on the other hand, signal angular acceleration of the head. The epithelium of the maculae and of the ampullary crests is composed of hair cells and supporting cells. Two types of hair cells are described — type I and type II. The base of a type I hair cell is

associated with a goblet-shaped nerve terminal belonging to the fast conducting afferent fibres of the vestibular nerve. The base of a type II hair cell, on the other hand, is either associated with a synaptic bouton of an afferent or efferent fibre of the vestibular nerve. The efferent fibres probably modify the threshold of the hair cells to sensory stimuli. A gelatinous mass, called an 'otolithic membrane', overlies each macula, and it contains crystalline bodies or otoliths. Alterations in the position of the head, relative to the line of gravity, are reflected in the drag of the otolithic membrane on the sensitive hair cells. A gelatinous dome-shaped mass called the 'cupula' rests on the surface of each ampullary crest. Currents in the endolymph swing the cupula from side to side, and stimulate the hair cells. Vestibular nerve fibres have a continuous basal discharge, and bending the cupula to one side will increase the frequency of discharge and to the opposite side will decrease the frequency (Fig. 4.19).

The epithelial lining of the uricle, saccule and semicircular ducts consist of light and dark cells. The cytoplasm of a dark cell contains numerous vesicles, mitochondria, lysosomes, granules and a prominent Golgi apparatus. These cells are therefore very active, and are said to be involved in the control of the ionic composition of the endolymph. The constitution of this fluid resembles intracellular fluid, being rich in potassium ions and low in sodium ions. In each ampulla there is a specialised epithelium on either side of the ampullary crest, called the 'planum semilunatum', and this is also thought to be concerned with the ionic composition of endolymph.

The cochlear duct is a spirally arranged tube concerned with hearing (Fig. 4.15). It starts below at the ductus reuniens and spirals above to a closed end near the apex of the cochlea. The floor is the basilar membrane which stretches from the spiral bony lamina to the spiral ligament of the outer wall of the cochlear canal. The roof is formed by the vestibular membrane, which also extends from the lamina to the outer surface of the cochlear canal. The cochlear duct is therefore triangular in cross-section. Above the attachment of the basilar membrane, the outer wall of the cochlear duct presents an external spiral sulcus, and above this is a spiral prominence. The epithelium above the promi-

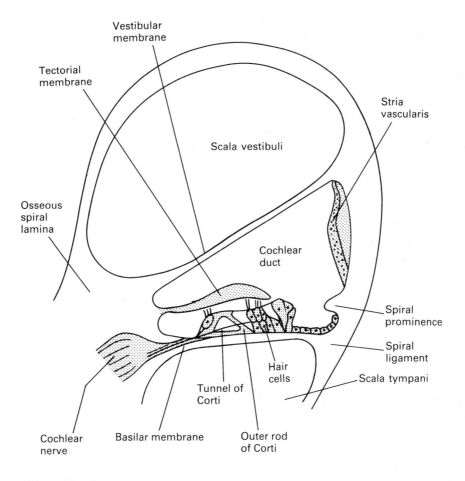

Fig. 4.15 Detail of the cochlear duct

nence is highly vascular and called the 'stria vascularis'. Like the dark cells and planum semilunatum it is also thought to be concerned with maintenance of the ionic composition of endolymph.

The specialised receptive organ for hearing lies in the cochlear duct on the basilar membrane, and is called the 'spiral organ of Corti'. The central part is composed of inner and outer rods of Corti. The cells have footplates which sit on the basilar membrane. The cells form pillars which slope towards each other to create a triangular tunnel of Corti. The sensitive hair cells are found on both the inner and outer sides of the pillars, and are therefore called 'inner' and 'outer hair cells' respectively. The outer hair cells are supported by phalangeal cells of Deiters and cells of Hensen.

The upper surfaces of the outer rods and Deiters' cells have flat phalangeal processes, which interdigitate to form a reticular membrane. Apart from the tunnel of Corti, there are other intercellular spaces between these cells. A space of Nuel is located between the outer rods of Corti and the outer hair cells, and an outer tunnel is found on the external side of the outer hair cells. These spaces contain a fluid called 'cortilymph', a fluid distinct from both endolymph and perilymph.

The basal poles of the inner and outer hair cells are in synaptic contact with both afferent and efferent fibres of the cochlear nerve. Like the efferent fibres of the vestibular nerve, these probably modulate transmission in the afferent fibres. The fibres from the outer hair cells pass across the canal of Corti and between the rods of Corti to join fibres from the inner hair cells. The combined fibres then pass through foramina in the osseous spiral lamina, their cell bodies lying within the spiral canal as the spiral ganglion. Central processes pass to the base of the cochlea in an osseous tunnel and finally through the internal acoustic meatus in the vestibulocochlear nerve. The membrana tectoria lies on the upper surface of the organ of Corti. It is composed of a jelly-like matrix, and the tips of the hair cell stereocilia are embedded in its undersurface. Vibrations in the basilar membrane vary with the intensity and frequency of the sound waves reaching it from the perilymph. Sheering forces are thus generated between the hair cells and the membrana tectoria. The type and intensity of distortion influences the rate of discharge and the number of discharging cochlear nerve fibres.

RADIOLOGY OF THE PETROUS TEMPORAL BONE

A certain amount of radiological information may be obtained from standard radiographs of the skull. Half axial and full axial views of the petrous temporal bone will show the internal acoustic meatus, the semicircular canals and cochlea. The internal acoustic meatus can also be shown on a frontal view, and the mouth of the internal acoustic meatus by using special projections. Oblique views of the mastoid region will show the mastoid process and its air cells. Computed tomography of the region, however, is the investigation of choice for detailed investigation of problems involving the petrous bone and the cerebellopontine angle. The cerebellopontine cistern is a lateral extension from the pontine cistern, and contains the 7th and 8th cranial nerves. A combination of cisternography and computed tomography is an excellent diagnostic procedure. Although positive contrast agents may be used for cisternography, it is often better to use air. A small mass in the cerebellopontine cistern will be outlined by this method.

EXAMINATION OF HEARING AND BALANCE

It is essential to perform simple clinical tests for the hearing threshold in every case of ear disease, no matter how minor. Such tests can give a rough estimate of the hearing threshold, and often differentiate between conductive and sensorineural deafness. The former type of deafness is a result of damage to the conducting mechanism which transmits sound from the external ear to the inner ear. Conduction abnormalities may therefore be caused by blockage of the external acoustic meatus, tympanic membrane damage, or disease of the middle ear ossicles. Sensorineural deafness is the result of disease of the cochlea, the cochlear part of the 8th nerve, or its central connections.

The voice test is the simplest way of assessing the hearing threshold. The subject is asked to occlude one ear, and the distance at which forced whispered sentences can be heard with the other ear is measured. Normally this is about 18 feet. If there is a degree of deafness in one ear, and it is necessary to raise the voice before it can be heard, the opposite ear must be masked. This is done by placing a Bárány noise box over the ear not under test. This box, driven mechanically, produces a noise. If, therefore, a subject cannot hear a loud shout with a box over the opposite ear, this is diagnostic of total deafness in the ear under test. Several tuning-fork tests may be used to determine whether deafness is of the conductive or the sensorineural type. The sound from a tuning-fork may be conducted to the cochlea through air and the normal sound-conducting pathways, or it may be transmitted through the bones of the skull. Conduction through the normal pathways is more efficient than bone conduction. In Rinne's test, the subject is asked to listen to the tuning-fork. With the fork still vibrating, the base is applied to the mastoid process and the patient asked which type of sound is louder. Normally, air-conducted sound is louder than bone-conducted sound (Fig. 4.16A). In this case, Rinne's test is said to be positive. If the sound-conducting pathway is damaged, however, bone conduction is better than air conduction, and the test is said to be negative (Fig. 4.16B). The test is not infallable however, because a total sensorineural deafness may appear to give a negative result. Although air conduction is absent, bone conduction is picked up because of sound being transmitted to the *opposite* cochlea (Fig. 4.17).

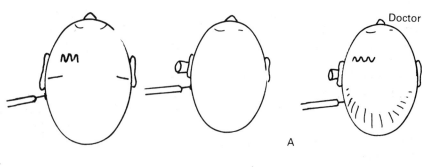

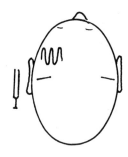

Fig. 4.18 Tuning fork tests — 3. A: Examiner-controlled test. B: Weber's test.

Fig. 4.16 Tuning fork tests — 1. A: Positive Rinne's test. B: Negative Rinne's test, conductive deafness.

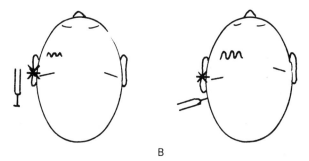

Fig. 4.17 Tuning fork tests — 2. A: Total left sensorineural deafness. B: False negative.

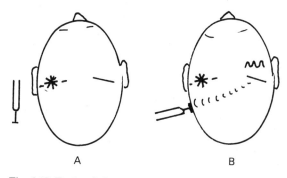

Bone conduction tests may also be made with the aid of a tuning-fork. The vibrating tuning-fork is placed on the mastoid process while the meatus is occluded, and the patient indicates when the sound disappears. The fork is immediately applied to the examiner's mastoid process with the meatus occluded (Fig. 4.18A). It is essential that the examiner has normal hearing for this test to be valid. If the examiner can still hear the tuning

fork, the patient's inner ear function is reduced, and bone conduction is said to be shortened. Weber's test is a bone conduction test which is especially sensitive for showing conductive deafness in one ear. The vibrating fork is placed on the vertex of the skull in the midline (Fig. 4.18B). The patient is asked if the sound is louder in one ear than the other or if it seems to be central. In unilateral conductive deafness the sound is heard louder in the affected ear. During examination, if Rinne's test has been negative in one ear, careful attention should be paid to Weber's test in order to exclude a false negative Rinne's test. The tests described can be performed by the student in a clinical situation, but further examination of hearing must be left to the specialist. An account of audiometry is outside the scope of this text.

Although highly specialised tests for vestibular function are available in special laboratories, the student can often make an initial assessment of vestibular function. Romberg's test is a simple way to examine balance. The patient is asked to stand with the feet together and the eyes closed. The subject will sway or fall to the side of a recent vestibular lesion. A patient with a vestibular disorder frequently complains of dizziness (vertigo) and often presents with nystagmus. 'Nystagmus' is a term which describes jerky movements of the eyes. Although there are other causes for the condition, vestibular nystagmus consists of a slow movement of the eyes, followed by a rapid return movement. Such nystagmus may be spontaneous, and immediately obvious on examination. It is usually most marked when the patient looks in the direction of the quick component. At other times nystagmus is only found in certain positions of the head. Sometimes nystagmus will not be evident, but may be induced and investigated by stimulation of the vestibular apparatus by rotational and caloric tests. The effects of angular rotation are best understood by considering the transverse canals (Fig. 4.19). Acceleration of the head to the right causes the endolymph to move to the left, and the cupula deflection is shown in the diagram.

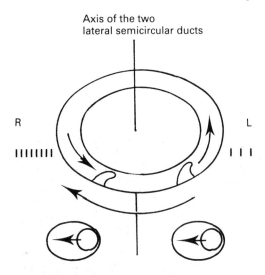

Axis of the two
lateral semicircular ducts

R   L

Fig. 4.19 Effects of rotation on the semicircular canals

Movement of endolymph towards the ampulla increases the impulse rate, and movement away from the ampulla decreases it. The difference in impulse rates is interpreted as a sensation of rotation, and the eyes move to the left. Once they have reached as far as they can, a central reflex quickly returns them to the midline. Thus there is nystagmus consisting of a slow vestibular movement followed by a rapid central movement. If

rotation suddenly stops, the endolymph moves to the right, and cupola deflection is to the right, although the semicircular canals are stationary. This signals a sensation of rotating to the left, even though the head is stationary. Nystagmus will then be easy to observe, and will consist of a slow component to the right followed by a rapid component. Damage to the vestibular apparatus or nerve will clearly have an effect on such tests. Rotational tests, however, have a limited clinical application, and a better way of stimulating each labyrinth separately is by syringing the ear with hot or cold water. Such caloric tests induce convection currents in the horizontal semicircular canals with resulting vertigo and nystagmus. In order to perform the test, the patient lies supine with the head bent forward at an angle of 30°. This brings the horizontal semicircular canal into a vertical plane. Cold fluid in the ear cools the most superficial part of the canal. The cooler endolymph falls, and causes movement away from the ampulla. A nystagmus results with the slow component going in the same direction as the fluid movement. Thus, stimulation of the left canal results in a slow component to the left with a fast component to the right. The patient complains of a sensation of rotation to the side of the test, and also of nausea. The response is measured as the number of seconds between the commencement of stimulation, and the cessation of nystagmus. Lesions in the vestibule or in the nerve result in depression of response or canal paresis. In addition to noting the response in time, the ease with which nystagmus is induced is documented.

CASES 4 AND 5

Valery Vixen and Gordon McNock were two patients with acoustic neuromas seen in the ear clinic. Unlike that of Mangla Mould, however, these neuromas were small, and were inside the internal acoustic meatus. In order to examine the internal acoustic meatus by CT, air was introduced into the cerebellopontine angle in both patients. Air failed to enter the internal acoustic meatus in Valery (Fig. 4.20). Some air did enter the meatus in Gordon, but showed a dilated meatus, which contained a tumour (Fig. 4.21). Both tumours were removed without facial nerve damage with the aid of a dissecting microscope.

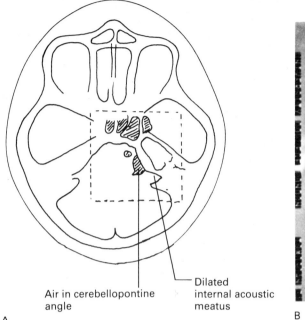

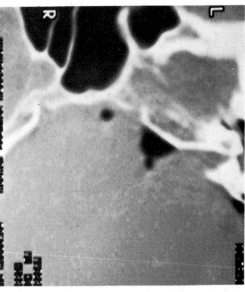

Air in cerebellopontine angle

Dilated internal acoustic meatus

A

B

Fig. 4.20 Valery Vixen. A: Tracing of CT scan. B: CT scan of head

Air in cerebellopontine angle

Tumour in internal acoustic meatus

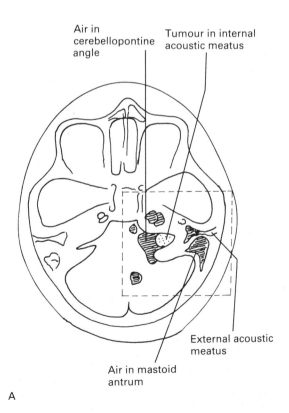

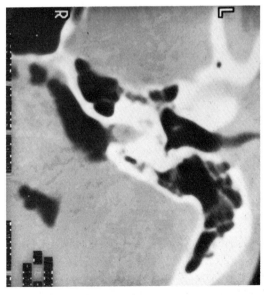

External acoustic meatus

Air in mastoid antrum

A

B

Fig. 4.21 Gordon McNock. A: Tracing of CT scan. B: CT scan of petrous temporal bone.

CASE 6

This subject was a male musician. He had complained of increasing deafness and buzzing in the ears since the age of 28. He had consulted several eminent physicians, including Franz Gerhard Wegeler. Some treatment was given, but by the age of 44 deafness had become severe, although he could still carry on some sort of a conversation with the aid of a speaking-tube. He had several severe illnesses during the next few years and died at the age of 56. A post-mortem was carried out by Johan Wagner and his assistant Rokitansky, during which the petrous temporal bones were removed for examination. The man was Ludwig van Beethoven, and his petrous temporal bones were placed in the Vienna Museum of Pathological Anatomy. Unfortunately they disappeared, and were said to have been sold to an English doctor. Several theories have been put forward about the cause of Beethoven's deafness. Perhaps the most likely is that he had otosclerosis. The bone immediately surrounding the membranous labyrinth is dense and fairly avascular. Outside this is lamella bone. The two are separated by a lymph space. In otosclerosis, the normal bone is absorbed and replaced by spongy vascular tissue. The stapes, in particular, becomes fixed. Nowadays, it is possible to remove the stapes and insert a prosthesis. Beethoven unfortunately benefited neither from a diagnosis nor appropriate treatment.

The student may find the anatomy of the petrous temporal bone and the ear difficult. It is knowledge, however, which should prove valuable no matter what specialty is eventually chosen. Problems with hearing and balance present in many patients, and the student should have an understanding of form and function of the ear, and be able to carry out the initial stages of investigation.

PART TWO

The Neck

5

BASIC TOPOGRAPHY OF THE NECK

The neck has anterior and posterior compartments. The anterior compartment is a tubular structure containing the pharynx, larynx, and neurovascular structures. The posterior compartment consists of the cervical vertebral column and its surrounding musculature, and is described in Chapter 1 of Volume 1.

The basic topography of the anterior compartment is simple. In the midline are *two tubes*, the larynx and trachea in front and the pharynx behind. It should be noted that the upper limit of the neck is the hyoid bone, structures belonging to the floor of the mouth occupying the space above, between the hyoid bone and mandible. This latter region is best studied with the mouth, and is therefore not included in this description of the neck. A further point needs to be made concerning the pharynx. When viewed from the side, it is overlapped by the angle of the mandible. In order therefore to get a complete view of the side of the neck, several structures belonging to the mouth need to be removed (Fig. 5.1). These include the ramus of the mandible and its musculature — temporalis, masseter, and pterygoids. The nerve to the facial muscles on the outside of the mandible also needs removal, together with the nerve on the inside of the mandible, the mandibular branch of the trigeminal nerve. Finally, the parotid gland will be removed. It is only in this way that the full extent of the pharynx is exposed from the base of the skull to the root of the neck. The styloid process and its three muscles — styloglossus, stylopharyngeus and stylohyoid — will also be revealed at the side of the pharynx.

On either side of the midline tubes are several

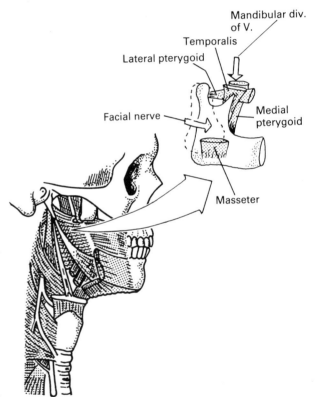

Fig. 5.1 The structures to be removed for the exposure of the upper pharynx

ascending and descending neurovascular structures (Fig. 5.2). These include the carotid tree, the internal jugular vein and several cranial nerves. There are passageways at both the upper and lower ends of the neck for these structures to leave and enter the region. At the upper end of the neck is a series of foramina in the base of the skull. Figure

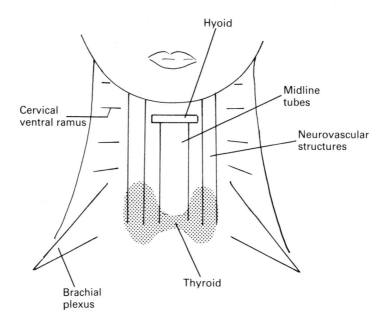

Fig. 5.2 Basic topography of the neck

5.3 shows the skull with these foramina labelled. From before back, these are the foramen ovale, foramen spinosum, carotid foramen, jugular foramen and the hypoglossal canal. The stylomastoid foramen is also shown in the diagram. The opening at the lower limit of the neck is the superior aperture of the thorax. The subclavian artery and vein pass through this aperture, and may be followed over the upper border of the 1st rib to the apex of the axilla and the upper limb. The thyroid gland clasps the front and sides of the larynx and trachea, and overlaps the carotid tree on either side.

A gap between the base of the skull and the atlas together with a series of intervertebral foramina are located lateral to the neurovascular structures. The *eight cervical ventral rami* emerge through these holes in the neck (Fig. 5.2). The upper four form a cervical plexus for supply of skin and muscle in the neck and thorax. The lower four, together with most of the ventral ramus of the 1st thoracic spinal nerve, form the brachial plexus for the supply of the upper limb. The ventral rami are closely related to the *scalene muscles* (Fig. 5.4). These three muscles arise from cervical vertebrae and

extend to the upper two ribs. Scalenus anterior arises from anterior tubercles of the mid-cervical vertebrae, and inserts below by a pointed tendon into a scalene tubercle on the inner border of the 1st rib. The scalenus medius arises from the axis and posterior tubercles of cervical vertebrae, and inserts into the 1st rib in front of its tubercle. A triangular gap is therefore formed, bounded by scalenus anterior, scalenus medius and the 1st rib, and is called the 'scalene triangle'. The trunks of the brachial plexus and the subclavian artery pass through the triangle. Indeed, the artery and the 1st thoracic ventral ramus groove the upper surface of the 1st rib. The scalenus posterior is small and deeply situated, and inserts into the 1st and 2nd ribs. Delicate *prevertebral muscles* are located in front of the cervical column. These, together with the scalene muscles, are covered with prevertebral fascia. The ventral rami thus lie deep to this layer of fascia. Indeed, as the subclavian artery and the trunks of the brachial plexus pass through the scalene triangle towards the apex of the axilla, they carry with them a prolongation of this fascia called the 'axillary sheath'.

The neck is described in this section using the

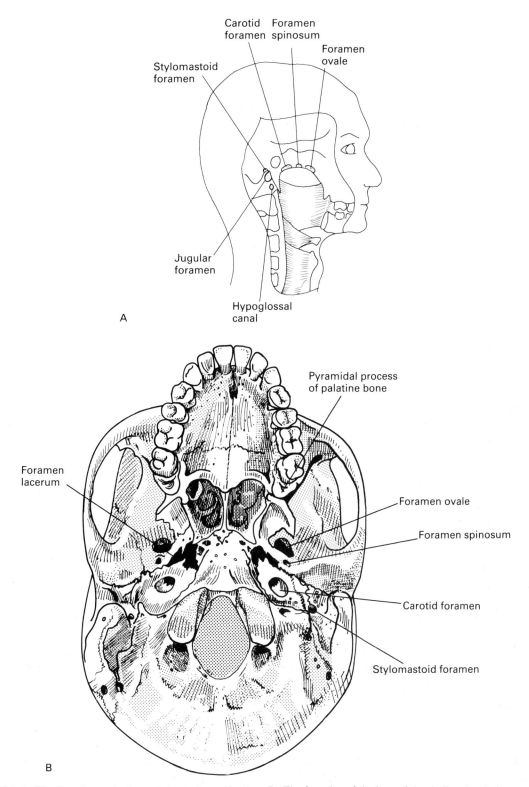

Fig. 5.3 A: The foramina at the base of the skull — side view. B: The foramina of the base of the skull — basal view.

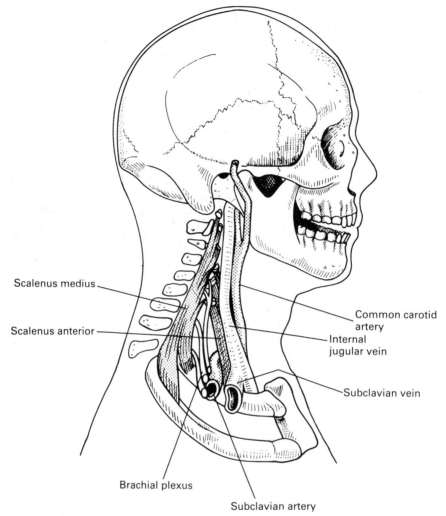

Scalenus medius

Scalenus anterior

Common carotid
artery

Internal
jugular vein

Subclavian vein

Brachial plexus

Subclavian artery

Fig. 5.4 The scalene triangle

pattern just outlined. Details are given in this chapter of the ascending and descending neuro-vascular structures. These include the carotid tree, subclavian tree, internal jugular vein and the 9th, 10th, 11th, and 12th cranial nerves. This is followed by a description of the cervical ventral rami and the cervical plexus. Finally, an outline of the superficial muscles, the investing layer of deep cervical fascia, and lymph nodes will be given. The larynx is dealt with in detail in Chapter 6, the pharynx in Chapter 7 and the thyroid in Chapter 8.

NEUROVASCULAR STRUCTURES

1. The carotid tree

The right and left common carotid arteries enter the neck behind their respective sternoclavicular joints. The right artery begins at the bifurcation of the brachiocephalic trunk, but the left artery is a direct branch of the aortic arch. Variations in origin, however, occur. The common carotid artery is surrounded in the neck by a sheath of loose connective tissue and this also invests the internal jugular vein and vagus nerve. The artery ends at

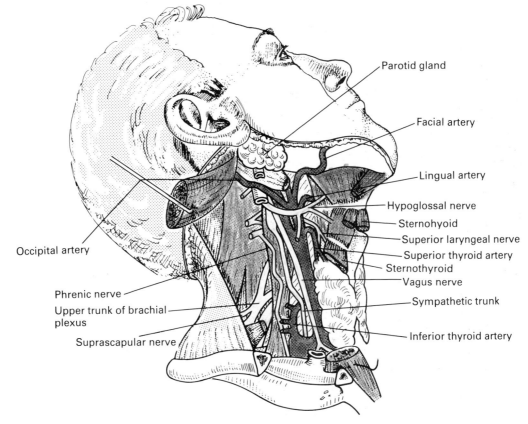

Fig. 5.5 The neurovascular structures of the neck

the upper border of the thyroid cartilage of the larynx by dividing into the external and internal carotid arteries. On rare occasions the division may occur at a higher or a lower level. The common carotid is dilated at the point where it bifurcates to form the carotid sinus, and specialised endings in the wall of this sinus are sensitive to changes in arterial blood pressure. A small chemoreceptor called the 'carotid body' is located just behind the point of division of the common carotid. There are usually no branches from the common carotid artery in the neck, but the student should always be prepared for variations in arterial pattern, and sometimes major arteries arise from the common carotid artery rather than from adjacent arteries.

The internal carotid artery may be traced upwards from its origin to the carotid foramen in the base of the skull. Its intracranial course is described in Chapter 2. In the neck, its course takes

it in front of the transverse processes of the upper three cervical vertebrae. Like the common carotid, it is also closely related to the internal jugular vein and vagus nerve, and enclosed with these structures in the carotid sheath. The internal carotid artery lies close to the wall of the pharynx during its ascent, being separated from it by a little fatty tissue and the ascending pharyngeal branch of the external carotid. The external carotid artery, at its origin, lies anterior and medial to the internal carotid. Traced upwards, however, it soon curls back to lie superficial to it. It ascends to a point behind the neck of the mandible, and here within the substance of the parotid gland, it divides into its terminal branches — the superficial temporal and maxillary arteries. Apart from these two terminal branches, it usually has six other branches (Fig. 5.5). These vessels will be described in subsequent chapters, but they may be listed at this point. The first branch, the *superior thyroid* artery, comes from the front of the external carotid and passes down to the upper pole of the thyroid lobe. The details of this vessel are given in Chapter 8. The *ascending pharyngeal* artery is a slender branch which also arises close to the origin of the external carotid. It ascends between the internal carotid artery and the side of the pharynx, and supplies branches to the constrictor muscles and the tonsil. On reaching the base of the skull it supplies meningeal branches which enter the cranial cavity through several foramina (foramen lacerum, jugular foramen and hypoglossal canal). In the region of the jugular foramen it also gives a branch which accompanies Jacobson's nerve into the tympanic cavity. The *lingual* artery, as its name implies, supplies the tongue and floor of the mouth. It arises opposite the tip of the greater cornu of the hyoid, and can be recognised by a characteristic loop which it makes before disappearing deep to the hyoglossus. The details of the lingual artery are given in Chapter 11. The *facial* artery arises at a higher level, medial to the ramus of the mandible. It grooves the submandibular gland, or passes through its substance, to reach the lower border of the mandible and the face. In the neck, the facial artery gives off an *ascending palatine* artery which ascends between styloglossus and stylopharyngeus to the side of the pharynx. Here it lies on the superior constrictor muscle outside the floor of the tonsillar fossa. It gives branches which, after piercing the superior constrictor, supply the palatine tonsil. Its branches anastomose with branches of the ascending pharyngeal artery. The *tonsillar* artery itself usually arises from the facial artery, and also pierces the superior constrictor to reach the tonsil. The course of the facial artery is described in Chapter 12. The *occipital and posterior auricular* arteries are branches which arise from the back of the external carotid, and both follow a course closely related to the posterior belly of digastric. The occipital artery runs along the lower border of the digastric and the posterior auricular along its upper border. The terminal branches of the external carotid, the *maxillary and superficial temporal* arteries, are described in Chapter 12.

2. The subclavian tree

The *subclavian* artery arises from the brachiocephalic trunk on the right, and directly from the aortic arch on the left. Descriptively the artery is divided into three parts by the scalenus anterior muscle (Fig. 5.6). The first part is the section of the artery between its origin and the medial border of scalenus anterior. The second part lies behind the muscle, and the third part extends from the lateral border of the muscle to the outer border of the 1st rib. The subclavian arteries arch over the suprapleural membranes, which in turn cover the domes of the pleura. Several important nervous structures are related to the subclavian arteries as they pass between the thorax and neck. The vagus nerve crosses the front of the first part of the artery on both sides. Tiny cardiac branches of both parasympathetic and sympathetic systems also stream over the front of the artery. On the left side, the phrenic nerve also lies close to the first part of the artery, but on the right side it is held away by the brachiocephalic vein and superior vena cava (see Fig. 8.3). The sympathetic trunk is located behind the first part of the subclavian artery on each side, and in particular, at the neck of the 1st rib is its stellate ganglion, when this is present. A loop of sympathetic tissue, the ansa subclavia, loops around the first part of the artery from the middle ganglion to the inferior or stellate ganglion (see Fig. 8.4). The right recurrent laryngeal nerve loops under the subclavian artery and then ascends in the tracheo-oesophageal groove. On the left, the nerve is already in the tracheo-oesophageal groove, having looped around the arch of the aorta. It is therefore only related to the thoracic part of the subclavian artery, and in the root of the neck lies deep in the tracheo-oesophageal groove. On the left side, the thoracic duct emerges from behind the oesophagus and passes upwards over the subclavian artery into the root of the neck where it arches forwards to the front of the artery to reach its destination.

The second part of the subclavian artery is hidden from view by the scalenus anterior. The third part of the artery is closely related to the lower trunk of the brachial plexus, while above it lie the middle and upper trunks of the plexus. The artery and plexus are crossed at the root of the neck by the inferior belly of the omohyoid and by the suprascapular and superficial cervical arteries. The small nerve to the subclavius descends in front of the third part of the artery.

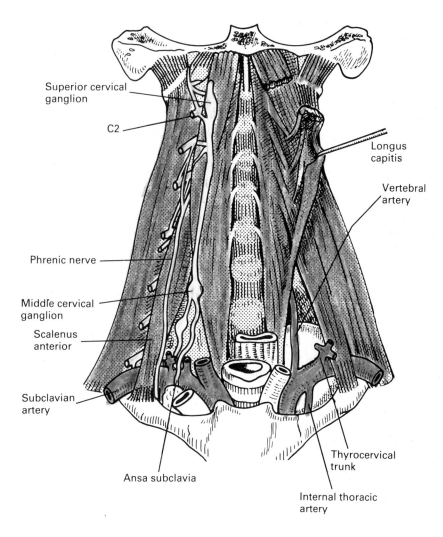

Fig. 5.6 The prevertebral region

As with other vessels in the neck, the student must be prepared to find variations in origin, course, and distribution of the branches of the subclavian artery. Typically, the branches arising from the first part of the artery are the vertebral artery, the internal thoracic artery and the thyrocervical trunk. The *vertebral* artery is a stout vessel which ascends to the transverse process of the 6th cervical vertebra. Here it enters the foramen transversarium and ascends through successive foramina until it reaches the upper surface of the atlas. On emerging from the foramen transversarium of the atlas, the vessel curves behind the lateral mass

with the ventral ramus of the 1st cervical nerve. It then dips under the posterior atlanto-occipital membrane, pierces both dura and arachnoid, and ascends in front of the spinal roots of the accessory nerve. It enters the cranial cavity through the foramen magnum and unites with its opposite number to form the basilar artery. Its intracranial course is described in Chapter 2. While in the neck, the vertebral artery gives spinal branches which reach the vertebral canal through the upper intervertebral foramina. During its course in the neck, the vertebral artery is accompanied by a plexus of veins which unite to form a single vertebral vein. This usually leaves the cervical spine through the foramen transversarium of the 7th cervical vertebra. Occasionally more than one vertebral vein will be found. In its ascent through successive foramina transversaria, the vertebral artery is also accompanied by a large sympathetic branch of the stellate ganglion.

The *internal thoracic* artery also arises from the first part of the subclavian artery. It descends into the thorax, and its course is described in Volume 3. The *thyrocervical trunk* is the third branch of the first part of the subclavian artery. It is a short vessel which arises close to the border of scalenus anterior. It usually divides into the inferior thyroid artery, suprascapular artery, and superficial cervical artery. The course of the inferior thyroid artery takes it *behind* the common carotid and carotid sheath to approach the thyroid lobe. Details of the course of this vessel are given in Chapter 8. Both suprascapular and superficial cervical arteries pass backwards in front of the scalenus anterior and phrenic nerve to reach the lower part of the posterior triangle of the neck. Here they lie superficial to the brachial plexus. The suprascapular artery usually passes above the superior transverse ligament of the scapula and supplies supraspinatus and infraspinatus. It also gives branches to surrounding muscles. The superficial cervical artery lies at a higher level and supplies muscles at the back of the posterior triangle of the neck.

The *costocervical trunk* is usually the only branch to arise from the second part of the subclavian artery. It arches backwards over the dome of the pleura to the neck of the 1st rib. Here it divides into a superior intercostal artery and a deep cervical artery. This latter branch supplies muscles around the cervical part of the vertebral column. The *dorsal scapular* artery is usually the only branch to arise from the third part of the subclavian artery. It weaves backwards through the brachial plexus in the floor of the posterior triangle of the neck to reach levator scapulae. Here it disappears from view and supplies adjacent muscles.

3. The internal jugular vein

The *internal jugular* vein begins in the jugular notch as a continuation of the sigmoid sinus, and here is dilated as the superior bulb of the jugular. It descends in the carotid sheath accompanied by the internal and common carotid arteries and the vagus nerve. It ends behind the sternal end of the clavicle by uniting with the subclavian vein to form a brachiocephalic vein. At its termination it is dilated into an inferior bulb, and just above this, the vein contains a pair of valves. The superior vena cava and brachiocephalic veins, on the other hand, are valveless. In its course in the carotid sheath it has the internal and common carotid arteries on its medial side. The surface anatomy of the internal jugular vein is important, because the vein may be used during central venous cannulation. Its upper end lies over the arch of the atlas, and its lower end deep to the triangle formed by the clavicle and the sternal and clavicular heads of sternocleidomastoid. Between these two points the vein is deep to sternocleidomastoid. The internal jugular vein receives various tributaries in the neck. The inferior petrosal sinus joins the superior bulb of the internal jugular. It receives veins from the face and tongue, and from the pharyngeal plexus of veins on the outer surface of the pharynx. It also receives superior and middle thyroid veins. Major lymph trunks also open into the venous system. The thoracic duct usually opens into the junction of the left internal jugular and subclavian veins. On the right side the right lymphatic duct usually opens into the veins at this junction. A pulsation from the internal jugular vein can sometimes be observed in the root of the neck, especially in cases of right atrial hypertrophy. Such a pulsation will be noted just before the corresponding carotid pulsation.

4. The subclavian vein

The *subclavian vein* starts at the outer border of the 1st rib in front of its corresponding artery and in front of the scalenus anterior (see Fig. 5.4). It does *not* therefore pass through the scalene triangle. It ends by uniting with the internal jugular vein to form the brachiocephalic vein. On the surface, its course can be represented by a convex line traced from the mid-clavicular point to the sternal end of the clavicle.

5. Central venous cannulation through the internal jugular and subclavian veins.

To reach the internal jugular vein, the patient is placed in a 20° head-down position. The right internal jugular is the preferred side because it is easier for a right-handed person and because there is no danger of damage to the thoracic duct. The subject's head is turned to the opposite side. A needle is attached to a saline-filled syringe, and with one hand palpating the carotid pulsation, it is inserted just lateral to the artery. The puncture is made through the centre of the triangle formed by the two heads of sternocleidomastoid and the clavicle (Fig. 5.7). The needle is inserted parallel to the midline, with the syringe raised to 30° above the skin. Gentle aspiration is applied to the syringe throughout the procedure, and there is a gush of blood into the syringe once the vein has been entered.

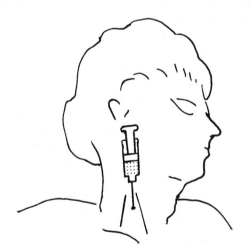

Fig. 5.7 Internal jugular vein cannulation

The subclavian vein may be approached from below or above the clavicle. For the infraclavicular approach, the patient is placed in a 20° head-down position. Once again, the right side is preferable, and the patient's head is turned to the opposite side. The needle is attached to a saline-filled syringe, and the mid-point of the clavicle and suprasternal notch identified. The needle is inserted below the mid-point of the clavicle and directed towards the suprasternal notch. The vein lies at some distance from the skin, and therefore a long needle is required. If gentle aspiration is maintained, a gush of blood enters the syringe when the vein is punctured. In the supraclavicular approach, the needle is placed in the angle between the clavicle and the clavicular head of sternocleidomastoid. The needle is directed towards the middle of the manubrium. The syringe is raised 15° above the skin. It should be noted that with this procedure, the tip of the needle is directed towards the dome of the pleura, and therefore it is much easier to injure this structure than with an infraclavicular approach. Indeed, the commonest complication of subclavian puncture is pneumothorax. A chest radiograph will indicate the degree of pneumothorax. Other complications include injury to the thoracic duct with a left puncture, injury to the brachial plexus, and injury to the phrenic nerve. Subclavian arterial damage may also occur if the artery is inadvertently entered. It must always be borne in mind that variations occur in the relationship of the subclavian vein to the clavicle, scalenus anterior, and 1st rib. The course of the subclavian vein also differs on right and left sides, and the course of the veins further changes if the head is tilted to one or other side. The position of the subclavian vein can, however, be accurately identified with the aid of a Doppler probe. If the ipsilateral arm is given a sharp squeeze, a typical venous hum indicates the position of the vein.

6. The glossopharyngeal, vagus, accessory and hypoglossal nerves in the neck

The 9th, 10th and 11th cranial nerves supply structures in the neck, but the 12th cranial nerve is a nerve of passage destined for the musculature of the tongue. In the neck, however, fibres from the 1st cervical ventral ramus hitch-hike along the hypoglossal nerve and leave it to supply musculature in the front of the neck.

The *glossopharyngeal nerve* enters the neck through the central part of the jugular foramen. It lies in a triangular depression in the petrous temporal bone, usually in its own sheath of dura. The glossopharyngeal nerve has superior and inferior sensory ganglia at its exit from the skull. The superior ganglion is very small, and found where the nerve lies in the pyramidal notch of the petrous temporal bone. The inferior ganglion lies at a lower level, below the jugular foramen. Sensory fibres for general sensation and taste have their cell bodies in these two ganglia. The nerve travels between the internal jugular vein and the internal carotid artery, deep to the styloid process, and reaches the stylopharyngeus muscle (Fig. 5.8). It enters the pharynx with this muscle through the gap between the superior and middle constrictors.

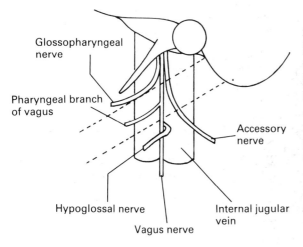

Fig. 5.8 The cranial nerves 9, 10, 11, and 12. The dotted line represents the posterior belly of the digastric.

The glossopharyngeal nerve has *communicating branches* just below the skull base. The nerve communicates with the superior cervical sympathetic ganglion of the sympathetic trunk, with the vagus, and with the auricular branch of the vagus. It also communicates with the facial nerve. The glossopharyngeal nerve gives its *tympanic branch (Jacobson's nerve)* just below the skull (see Ch. 4). This branch carries sensory fibres for the middle ear and auditory tube, and also parasympathetic fibres destined for the lesser petrosal nerve. This latter nerve carries its secretomotor fibres to the otic ganglion where, after synapse, they supply the parotid gland. In the neck, the glossopharyngeal nerve gives a *carotid* branch which descends on the internal carotid artery to the carotid sinus and carotid body. During its descent the nerve also receives vagal fibres. Before entering the pharynx, the glossopharyngeal nerve gives a *muscular branch*

to the stylopharyngeus. It also sends *pharyngeal branches* which join the pharyngeal plexus, and carry sensory fibres to the mucous membrane of the oral part of the pharynx. Once inside the pharynx, the nerve gives its *lingual branches* to supply the posterior third of the tongue with general and special sensation, a supply which includes the vallate papillae. The course of the nerve ends with *tonsillar branches*. These supply sensation to the tonsillar mucous membrane in a plexus of nerves with the posterior and middle palatine nerves.

The *vagus nerve* leaves the skull through the middle part of the jugular foramen. While in the jugular foramen it bears a superior ganglion, and soon after leaving the foramen has an inferior ganglion. Both ganglia contain sensory cell bodies. In the jugular fossa the superior ganglion gives off an *auricular branch (Arnold's nerve)*, and a *meningeal branch*. Descriptions of these nerves are given in Chapters 4 and 2 respectively. The cell bodies in the inferior ganglion are concerned with general visceral afferent input from many viscera from the larynx to the descending colon. The ganglion also contains a few cell bodies concerned with taste from the epiglottis and vallecula. Below the skull the vagus nerve has several *communicating branches*. Twigs from the superior ganglion connect the vagus to the glossopharyngeal nerve and the sympathetic trunk. Through the auricular branch, there is a communication with the facial nerve, and the significance of this communication is described in Chapter 4. Connections also exist between the inferior ganglion and the sympathetic trunk and the hypoglossal nerve. The *cranial part of the accessory nerve* blends with the vagus at the level of the inferior ganglion.

Below the jugular fossa the vagus descends within the carotid sheath between the internal carotid artery and internal jugular vein, and then between the common carotid artery and jugular vein (Figs. 5.8, 5.9). In the root of the neck, the right vagus passes in front of the first part of the subclavian artery and enters the thorax. On the left side, the vagus enters the thorax between the left subclavian artery and the left common carotid artery. While in the neck, both vagus nerves give *pharyngeal and laryngeal nerves*, and twigs which join the carotid branch of the glossopharyngeal nerve. The *pharyngeal branch of the vagus* is the

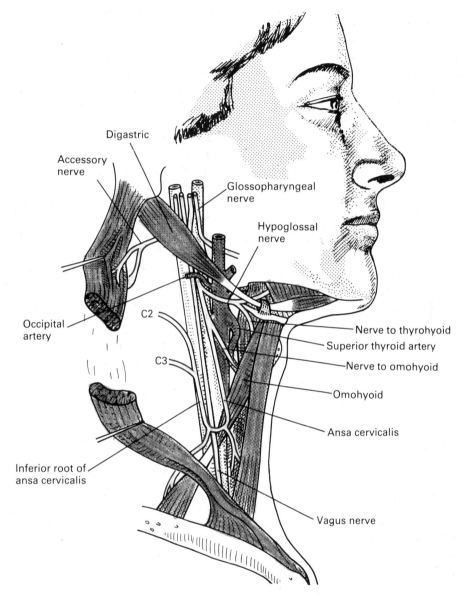

Digastric

Accessory
nerve

Glossopharyngeal
nerve

Hypoglossal
nerve

Occipital
artery

C2

C3

Nerve to thyrohyoid

Superior thyroid artery

Nerve to omohyoid

Omohyoid

Ansa cervicalis

Inferior root of
ansa cervicalis

Vagus nerve

Fig. 5.9 Details of the ansa cervicalis

main motor supply to the pharyngeal muscles. It consists mostly of cranial accessory fibres, and arises high on the vagus at the inferior ganglion. It descends between internal and external carotid arteries to the middle constrictor of the pharynx. Here it takes part in the formation of the pharyngeal plexus. It supplies the muscles of the pharynx with the exception of stylopharyngeus and cricopharyngeus, and muscles of the palate with the exception of tensor veli palatini. The *superior laryngeal nerve* also arises high on the vagus at the inferior ganglion. It descends along the side of the pharynx and divides into internal and external laryngeal nerves. The *recurrent laryngeal nerve* only arises from the cervical part of the vagus on the right side. It loops under the right subclavian artery and ascends obliquely to the tracheo-oesophageal groove. The left nerve emerges from the vagus in the thorax, passes behind the attachment of the ligamentum arteriosum to the arch of the aorta, and ascends in the tracheo-oesophageal groove. Details of the laryngeal nerves are given in Chapters 6 and 8. *Cardiac branches* arise from the vagus in the neck. There are usually two on each side, a superior and an inferior branch, and they descend to the cardiac plexuses.

The *accessory nerve* arises by two roots — a cranial root and a spinal root. The two roots unite for a while, but separate as they pass through the jugular foramen. The cranial fibres merge with the vagus nerve at its inferior ganglion, and are distributed through its pharyngeal and laryngeal branches. The intracranial course of the spinal root is described in Chapter 2. After leaving the jugular foramen, the spinal root passes backwards across the internal jugular vein (Fig. 5.8). It may, however, pass behind the vein, and in rare instances has even been found passing through the vein. The nerve reaches the deep surface of sternocleidomastoid, pierces the muscle and supplies it. Here, it is joined by branches of the 2nd and 3rd cervical ventral rami, which are said to be proprioceptive fibres. The accessory nerve emerges from the muscle and passes across the prevertebral fascial floor of the posterior triangle of the neck (Fig. 5.10). It lies on the fascia which covers levator scapulae, where it receives further communicating branches from the 3rd and 4th cervical ventral rami, also thought to be proprioceptive in nature. The nerve then enters and supplies trapezius.

The *hypoglossal nerve* is a nerve of passage in the neck, for it supplies motor fibres to the tongue. It emerges through the anterior condylar (hypoglossal) canal, deep to the internal jugular vein, and descends to the interval between the internal carotid and internal jugular vein (Figs. 5.8, 5.9). As it emerges from between these two vessels, it turns around the origin of the external carotid and the loop of the lingual artery to reach the floor of the mouth, deep to mylohyoid. The details of the hypoglossal nerve are given in Chapter 11. In the neck, however, it has important communicating fibres which reach it from the *1st cervical ventral ramus*. These hitch-hike along the nerve for a short distance and then leave it to supply geniohyoid and thyrohyoid, and form the upper root of the ansa cervicalis.

7. Cervical ventral rami

The upper four ventral rami of the cervical nerves unite in a plexiform manner as the *cervical plexus*. The lower four, together with most of the ventral ramus of the first thoracic nerve, form the *brachial plexus*. The brachial plexus is fully described in Chapter 9, Volume 1. The ventral ramus of the 1st cervical spinal nerve emerges above the posterior arch of the atlas, and that of the 2nd nerve between the atlas and axis (see Fig. 5.6). The 3rd and 4th ventral rami enter the neck through their respective intervertebral foramina. All four ventral rami supply twigs to prevertebral and adjacent muscles and communicate with each other to form a plexus on scalenus medius and levator scapulae. Communicating branches, sensory and motor branches arise from this cervical plexus. Communicating branches connect the upper two cervical ventral rami with the hypoglossal and vagus nerves, and with the sympathetic trunk. Cutaneous branches emerge at the posterior border of the sternocleidomastoid where they radiate to the skin on the side of the temple, the neck and upper thorax (Fig. 5.10). The *lesser occipital nerve* curls around the accessory nerve to reach the posterior border of sternocleidomastoid. It ascends to the back of the ear where it supplies skin on the side of the head and the upper part of the cranial surface of the auricle. The *great auricular nerve* is a large branch which ascends on the surface of the sternocleidomastoid in company with the external jugular vein. It reaches the surface of the parotid gland where it divides into anterior and posterior branches. The anterior branch is distributed to skin over the parotid gland itself, and the posterior branch supplies skin on the back of the ear and the lobule of the ear. The nerve is at risk during operations on the parotid gland (see Ch. 12). The *transverse cutaneous nerve of the neck* passes horizontally on the sternocleidomastoid to supply skin on the anterolateral aspect of the neck. *Supraclavicular nerves* arise from a common trunk, and descend over the clavicle to the upper part of the chest wall. They are usually described as being 'medial', 'intermediate' and 'lateral' in position.

Apart from *muscular twigs to prevertebral muscles*, the cervical plexus furnishes two other muscular branches, the *inferior root of the ansa cervicalis* and the *phrenic nerve*. The inferior root of the ansa is

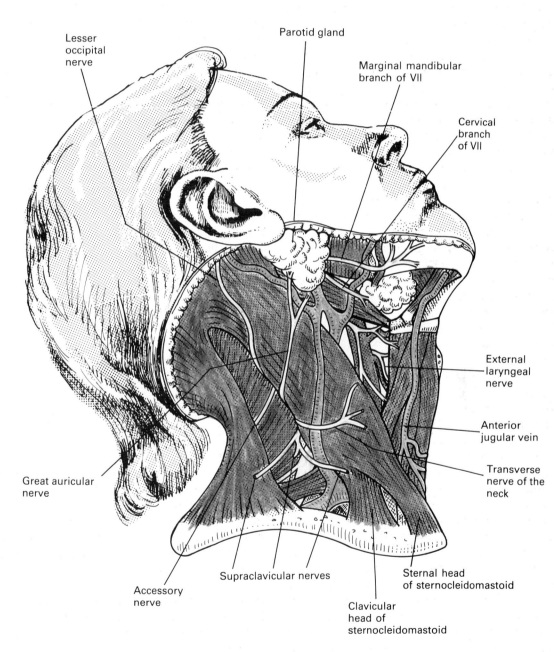

Lesser
occipital
nerve

Parotid gland

Marginal mandibular
branch of VII

Cervical
branch
of VII

External
laryngeal
nerve

Anterior
jugular vein

Transverse
nerve of the
neck

Great auricular
nerve

Accessory
nerve

Supraclavicular nerves

Clavicular
head of
sternocleidomastoid

Sternal head
of sternocleidomastoid

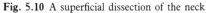

Fig. 5.10 A superficial dissection of the neck

usually formed from branches of the 2nd and 3rd cervical ventral rami (Fig. 5.9). It descends on the lateral side of the internal jugular vein and then loops upwards to join the superior root. This latter nerve, which comes from the hypoglossal nerve, lies on the common carotid artery. The loop so formed — the ansa cervicalis — supplies strap muscles at the front of the neck. The phrenic nerve, the only motor supply to the diaphragm, arises from the 3rd, 4th and 5th cervical ventral rami (see Fig. 5.6). It lies *behind* the prevertebral fascia on the anterior surface of scalenus anterior. The nerve crosses the obliquity of the muscle, bringing it in front of the subclavian artery, where it enters the thorax. The phrenic nerve not only contains motor fibres for the diaphragm but also many sensory fibres, which come from peritoneum, pleura and pericardium. Occasionally, an accessory phrenic nerve arises from the nerve to the subclavius, and this descends to the thorax in company with the main phrenic nerve and usually joins it somewhere in the thorax.

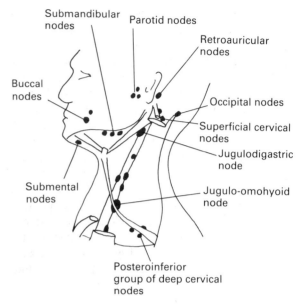

Fig. 5.11 Lymph nodes in the neck

8. Lymph nodes

Lymph from the head and neck drains into a group of lymph nodes closely associated with the carotid sheath. This deep cervical group receives lymph from structures of the head and neck either directly or indirectly after passing through regional groups of nodes. Several well demarcated groups are concerned with the initial drainage of the superficial tissues of the head and neck (Fig. 5.11). Occipital lymph nodes are found in the upper angle of the posterior triangle of the neck. A further group is found in front of this on the surface of the mastoid process at the back of the ear. These form the retroauricular group. Several superficial nodes are closely related to the parotid gland. They lie either outside or inside the parotid fascial covering. Some deep parotid nodes are placed within the substance of the gland. A buccal set of nodes is closely associated with the facial artery in the cheek. Below the angle and body of the mandible, three submandibular lymph nodes will be found. These are closely related to the facial artery and submandibular gland under the mandible. The submental lymph nodes lie under

the mylohyoid, between the anterior bellies of the digastric under the point of the chin. Several nodes are associated with the superficial jugular veins; the anterior cervical group lies close to the anterior jugular vein and the superficial cervical group is found along the external jugular vein. Some regional nodes are deeply placed. A retropharyngeal set of nodes lies between the pharynx and the prevertebral fascia. The nodes lie in the midline and laterally on either side. Paratracheal nodes lie on either side of the trachea. Infrahyoid, prelaryngeal and pretracheal nodes are located deep to the investing cervical fascia in front of the hyoid, larynx and trachea.

The deep cervical lymph nodes lie along the carotid sheath, and may be divided into superior and inferior groups. The superior group lies, for the most part, deep to sternocleidomastoid. One of these nodes is particularly large, and lies in a triangle bounded by the posterior belly of the digastric, the facial vein and the internal jugular vein. It is called the 'jugulodigastric' node. It is usually associated with one or two smaller lymph nodes, and is concerned with lymph drainage from the tongue and tonsil. The inferior group of deep cervical nodes lies deep to the lower part of sterno-cleidomastoid, and extends around the brachial plexus and subclavian vessels. One node in this group lies close to the intermediate tendon of the omohyoid and is called the 'jugulo-omohyoid' lymph node. It is especially concerned with lymph drainage from the tongue. Lymph ducts from the deep cervical nodes form a jugular trunk on each side of the neck. On the right side, the trunk usually ends by joining the junction of the internal jugular and subclavian veins. It may, however, join the right lymphatic duct. On the left side, it usually enters the thoracic duct, but other patterns of termination may be found. The student should pay particular attention to the position of the superficial and deep cervical lymph nodes. Examination of the head and neck should always include a careful palpation for enlarged lymph nodes.

CASE 1

Ethne Stonehenge, a 40-year-old computer sales-person, had been treated for a cancer of the tongue. Two years after the treatment she presented with several hard deep lymph nodes and a small superficial cervical node on the right. Biopsy of the superficial node showed that she had metastases from the cancer. A decision was made to remove the nodes surgically. Nodes in the neck are removed in a block of tissue which includes the sternocleidomastoid, deep cervical fascia, and the internal jugular vein and carotid sheath.

Operation notes and discussion
Considerable thought was given to the incision. Transverse incisions, along Langer's lines, heal well in the neck, and give a good cosmetic result. Vertical incisions, on the other hand may form fibrotic scars which bowstring. If vertical incisions are used, it is therefore better to follow a sinuous curve rather than a straight line. The planning of the skin flaps are particularly important, because if the blood supply of a flap edge is poor the wound breaks down after operation. The carotid tree, devoid of its coverings, will then be exposed. Blood supply to the skin of the neck comes from blood vessels which travel vertically down from the facial and submandibular regions on the one hand, and upwards from the supraclavicular and suprascapular regions on the other. With these points in mind, a transverse incision was made at this watershed between the upper two-thirds and lower third of the neck.

During removal of the block of tissue, precautions were taken against damage to nerves in the neck. In the upper part of the wound, the marginal mandibular branch of the facial nerve was carefully preserved (see Fig. 5.10). The nerve was found leaving the parotid gland just in front of the retromandibular vein. Its course was then followed *below* the mandible onto the surface of the submandibular gland. An incision into the fascia over the gland enabled the fascia and nerve to be retracted while the gland was being removed. The cervical branch of the facial nerve was sacrificed. During removal of the submandibular gland, the hypoglossal and lingual nerves were carefully avoided. The hypoglossal nerve was easily identified as it crossed the loop of the lingual artery, and it was traced deep to the gland. Care was taken when pulling on the gland not to pull the lingual nerve into the operative field.

During dissection in the region of the posterior triangle of the neck, the accessory nerve was found leaving the posterior border of the sternocleidomastoid and traced from here through the muscle. Once fully exposed, the sternocleidomastoid was removed from around it. Damage to the accessory nerve is one of the drawbacks of radical neck dissection. Unfortunately, sometimes the nerve is involved with lymph node disease, and then has to be sacrificed. During removal of the sternocleidomastoid, the cutaneous branches of the cervical plexus, the lesser occipital, great auricular, transverse nerve of neck and supraclavicular nerves were removed. The anaesthesia of the skin of the neck which this inevitably produces is usually well-tolerated by most patients. The phrenic nerve was not injured, because the prevertebral fascia covering scalenus anterior was not incised. The nerve could be seen behind this fascia on the surface of the muscle. Similarly, the brachial plexus was also left undisturbed by staying outside the prevertebral fascia.

During removal of the internal jugular vein, the vagus nerve was carefully preserved. The lymph nodes were not adherent to the carotid sheath. The sympathetic trunk, at the back of the carotid sheath, was also left undisturbed. In the lower part of the dissection care was taken not to injure the junction of the internal jugular and subclavian veins with the major lymph trunks. The pleural dome was not injured.

Ethne made a good recovery from the operation, but had recurrent metastases 18 months after the operation. In spite of further treatment, she died a few months later.

MUSCULOFASCIAL COVERING OF THE NECK

The *platysma* is a broad sheet of muscle in the sub-cutaneous fat at the front of the neck. Its fibres arise from the fascia over pectoralis major and del-toid and sweep upwards over the clavicle into the neck, many interdigitating across the midline. Above, some fibres insert into the mandible while others cross the mandible to gain insertion into the skin of the lower face. The platysma may be re-garded as a muscle of facial expression, and is sup-plied by the cervical branch of the facial nerve. When it contracts, it wrinkles the skin on the side of the neck and assists in drawing the angles of the mouth downwards.

Two large muscles, the *sternocleidomastoid* and *trapezius* lie on a plane deep to the platysma, and can be used to divide the neck into two large tri-angles (Fig. 5.12). In front is the large anterior triangle and on either side of the neck are the smaller posterior triangles. The structures between the hyoid bone and the mandible are classified in this book as belonging to the floor of the mouth rather than to the neck. For this reason the defi-nition of the boundaries of the anterior triangle of the neck differs from that given in most textbooks. The boundaries of the triangle are here defined as the anterior borders of the sternocleidomastoids on either side with a U-shaped base above of the di-gastrics and hyoid bone. The boundaries of the posterior triangle are clavicle below, and sterno-cleidomastoid and trapezius above. There is very little justification for descriptions which further subdivide these triangles. The only useful div-isions are anterior, posterior and scalene triangles. The anterior triangle of the neck contains the lar-ynx and thyroid, with parts of the carotid trees, jugular veins and associated nerves (see Fig. 5.10). The posterior triangle contains the cervical and brachial plexuses, and the accessory nerve. A fairly thick layer of deep cervical fascia invests the tra-pezius, forms the roof of the posterior triangle, in-vests the sternocleidomastoid muscle, and extends across the anterior triangle. It is attached above to both the hyoid bone and the mandible. Near the angle of the mandible the fascia splits to enclose the parotid gland. At the root of the neck this in-vesting layer of fascia is attached to the acromion,

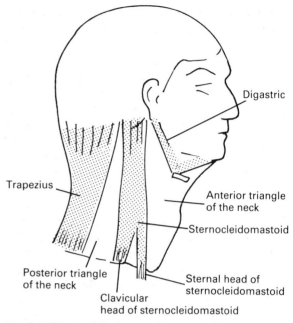

Fig. 5.12 The 'useful' triangles of the neck

the clavicle and the manubrium. In the supraster-nal notch, however, it splits into two layers, one layer attaching to the anterior border of the ma-nubrium and the other to the posterior border. There is thus a small suprasternal space between these two layers, containing a little fat, a lymph node, the lower sections of the anterior jugular veins, and the jugular venous arch. In the lower part of the posterior triangle a similar situation is found, for here the fascia also divides into two lamellae, the deeper of the two surrounding the in-ferior belly of omohyoid.

The *sternocleidomastoid* has two heads of origin. The sternal head is tendinous and arises from the front of the manubrium, and the clavicular head is muscular and arises from the medial third of the clavicle. Between these two heads of origin is a triangular gap filled by deep cervical fascia. The two heads of origin unite to form a thick muscle which inserts along a line extending from the mas-toid process to the lateral half of the superior nuchal line. Acting alone, the sternocleidomastoid approximates the mastoid process to the manu-brium and medial end of the clavicle. If you perform this action, you will find that the head has been rotated so that the face looks towards the opposite side and upwards. The sternocleidomastoids often assist other neck muscles in turning the head horizontally from side to side. Such movements are commonly seen in the spectators at a tennis match. Acting together, the two muscles draw the head forwards, the type of movement used in looking over someone's shoulder in a crowd. Sternocleidomastoid gains its motor supply from the spinal part of the accessory nerve. It also receives a rich proprioceptive supply from the 2nd and 3rd cervical ventral rami. Proprioceptive information from the neck muscles allows continuous assessment and readjustment of tone and position. Spasm of sternocleidomastoid is called torticollis. The head is held in a characteristic position with the face turned upwards to the side opposite the affected muscle. This sometimes occurs spontaneously in adults or may be associated with infected cervical lymph nodes in children.

The *trapezius* is a flat, triangular muscle lying over the back of the neck and upper thorax. Above, the muscle arises from the medial third of the superior nuchal line, the external occipital protuberance and the ligamentum nuchae. Traced downwards, it arises from the tip of the 7th cervical vertebra, and the supraspinous ligaments and spines of all the thoracic vertebrae. The fibres converge to the lateral third of the clavicle, the acromion, the crest of the scapula and to the tubercle of the spine of the scapula. The muscle is supplied by the accessory nerve. Branches from the 3rd and 4th cervical ventral rami provide proprioceptive fibres. Trapezius is mainly concerned with shoulder movement, and is described in more detail in Chapter 3 of Volume 1. With the shoulder fixed, however, it can draw the head backwards and laterally. Clinical testing of the spinal part of the accessory nerve involves testing the function and strength of both sternocleidomastoid and trapezius. Each sternocleidomastoid is tested by asking the subject to push the chin away from the side under test against the examiner's hand. Trapezius is tested by asking the subject to shrug the shoulders, and the strength can be gauged if the examiner rests his hands on the subject's shoulders.

The *infrahyoid strap muscles* are located at the front of the neck, on a plane deep to the investing layer of deep cervical fascia. The most superficial of these muscles is the *sternohyoid* (see Fig. 5.5). This arises from the back of the medial end of the clavicle and the manubrium, and ascends in front of the neck to its insertion into the body of the hyoid. In the lower part of the neck the sternohyoids are widely separated from each other, but they converge as they reach the hyoid. Deep to the sternohyoid is a shorter muscle, the *sternothyroid*. This pair of muscles, arising from the back of the manubrium, lie close together at their origins, but diverge as they pass to their insertions on the oblique lines of the thyroid cartilage. A small quadrilateral *thyrohyoid muscle* arises from the oblique line of the thyroid lamina, on each side, and ascends to the body and greater cornu of the hyoid bone. The *omohyoid* has two bellies. The inferior belly arises from the upper border of the scapula, crosses the lower part of the posterior triangle of the neck, and gives way to an intermediate tendon, deep to sternocleidomastoid (see Fig. 5.9). This tendon is held in place by a band of deep fascia which is attached below to the clavicle and 1st rib. Once through this loop of fascia, the intermediate tendon gives rise to the superior belly, which ascends to its insertion into the body of the hyoid bone. The infrahyoid strap muscles are all supplied by ventral rami of cervical nerves. Thyrohyoid receives its nerve supply from C1 fibres which have hitch-hiked for a short distance along the hypoglossal nerve. Omohyoid is supplied by the superior ramus of the ansa cervicalis and the ansa loop itself. Sternohyoid and sternothyroid are also supplied by the ansa cervicalis. The infrahyoid strap muscles, with the exception of sternothyroid, act on the hyoid bone, and these actions are described in more detail in Chapter 11. Those infrahyoid muscles which are inserted into the larynx, namely sternothyroid and thyrohyoid, are extrinsic muscles of the larynx. The sternothyroid is capable of drawing the larynx downwards, and the thyrohyoid can raise the larynx.

6

THE LARYNX

1. The cartilages and joints

The larynx is composed of several cartilages united by synovial joints, ligaments, and membranes. It has outer and inner walls which spring from a base made by the cricoid ring. The thyroid cartilage with the thyrohyoid membrane and the anterior cricothyroid ligament form the outer wall (Figs. 6.1, 6.2). The inner wall is made of the arytenoid cartilages, membrane and muscle (see Figs. 6.3, 6.5). The thyroid cartilage is the largest cartilage and consists of two laminae which meet in the midline at an angle of about 90° in men, and 120° in women. The size and shape of the larynx is similar in both male and female until puberty, but in the male there is a considerable increase in size and alteration in shape at puberty. The thyroid cartilage projects as a laryngeal prominence, and this may be seen and palpated in the midline of the neck. It is particularly obvious in the male, and is often called 'Adam's apple'. A thyroid notch may be palpated between the two laminae of

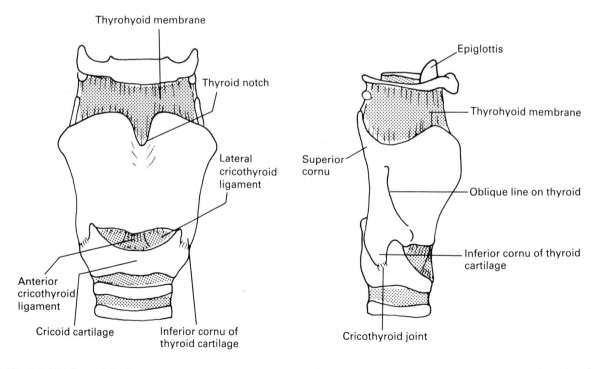

Fig. 6.1 The front of the larynx

Fig. 6.2 The side of the larynx

the thyroid cartilage above the laryngeal prominence. The posterior borders of the thyroid cartilage extend above and below as slender superior and inferior cornua.

The cricoid cartilage is said to have the shape of a signet ring, the narrow part lying in front, and the thick section behind. The anterior arch of the cricoid can be palpated in the living neck below the thyroid cartilage. The inferior cornu of each thyroid lamina articulates with a small facet on the side of the cricoid arch at a synovial articulation. The capsule of each cricothyroid joint is strong, especially posteriorly.

The outer wall of the larynx is completed by several membranes. The upper border of each lamina of the thyroid cartilage gives attachment to the thyrohyoid membrane, which stretches upwards *behind* the body and greater cornu of the hyoid to gain attachment to the back of the bone. There is often a bursa between the body of the bone and the membrane. The membrane is thickened in the midline as a median thyrohyoid ligament, and the edges are likewise thickened as the lateral thyrohyoid ligaments. The lower border of the thyroid cartilage is attached to the cricoid in the midline

by the strong anterior cricothyroid ligament. The lower border of the cricoid is attached to the uppermost ring of the trachea by the cricotracheal ligament.

The inner wall of the larynx is best appreciated by removing a thyroid lamina (Fig. 6.3). The leaf-like epiglottis, made of elastic fibrocartilage, is attached by the thyroepiglottic ligament to the angle of the thyroid laminae. It projects upwards behind the thyrohyoid membrane, hyoid bone and tongue. Paired arytenoid cartilages are located on the upper border of the lamina of the cricoid. Each cartilage is pyramidal in shape, having a base, three surfaces, and an apex. The joint between each arytenoid base and cricoid is synovial. The capsule of each joint is strong, especially posteriorly where it is thickened as a cricoarytenoid ligament. The inner wall of the larynx is completed by membrane which extends from the sides of the epiglottis to the arytenoids and down to the cricoid. The part of this fibroelastic membrane between the side of the epiglottis and arytenoid is called the quadrangular membrane. It is particularly well defined in its lower reaches, and ends as a free lower border between the arytenoid and the

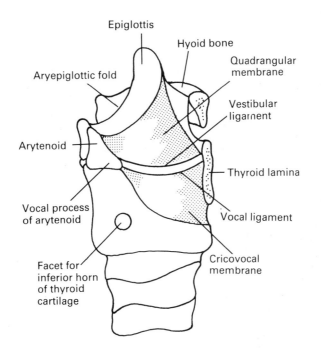

Fig. 6.3 The side of the 'inner tube'. The right thyroid lamina has been removed.

thyroid lamina. This free edge is called the *vestibular ligament*. The upper part of the quadrangular membrane is far less well developed, and is replaced by aryepiglottic muscle fibres. There is a slit-like gap in the fibroelastic inner wall below the vestibular ligament, but lower down, the wall is completed by the cricovocal membrane (lateral cricothyroid ligament). Each membrane is attached to the cricoid, and ends as a free upper border extending between the anterior point of the arytenoid and the angle between the two thyroid laminae. This upper, thickened free edge of the membrane is called the 'vocal ligament'. Because of the attachment of this important ligament to the anterior angle of the arytenoid, this point on the cartilage is referred to as the 'vocal process'. The anterior midline part of the cricovocal membrane, between the cricoid and thyroid cartilages, is called the anterior cricothyroid ligament.

The thyroid, cricoid and most of the arytenoid cartilages are made of hyaline cartilage. They tend to ossify from the mid-twenties, and in later life may be completely ossified. Ossification is often evident on radiographs of the neck as irregular opacities in the cartilages. The epiglottis, apices of the arytenoids, corniculate and cuneiform cartilages are made of elastic fibrocartilage.

The larynx is an organ of ·phonation, and a sphincteric air passage. It also protects the tracheobronchial tree. If this protective role is deranged, laryngeal incompetence results, and food and fluid may be aspirated into the trachea. The structures involved in the production of sound and in regulation of the airway size are the vocal ligaments. It is therefore important to understand how movements at the cricothyroid and cricoarytenoid joints produce changes in tension and position of the ligaments. Movement occurs at the two crico-thyroid joints around an axis which passes transversely through both joints. A movement at the cricothyroid joints which tilts the thyroid cartilage forwards will increase the distance between the vocal processes of the arytenoids and the thyroid angle, and will result in an increase in tension of the vocal ligaments. If the cricoid tilts relative to the thyroid, by a movement which draws up the arch of the cricoid and tilts back the cricoid lamina, tension will also increase in the vocal ligaments. Movements at the cricothyroid joints are therefore responsible for changes in *tension* in the vocal ligaments. Movements at the cricoarytenoid joints are more complex (Fig. 6.4). The cartilages can be abducted away from the laryngeal midline or adducted towards it. In addition rotational movements are said to occur through an almost vertical axis, and these also take the vocal processes away from and towards the midline. Thus the gap between the vocal ligaments, the rima glottidis, alters in both size and shape with abduction and adduction of the ligaments. Figure 6.4A shows the arytenoids and vocal ligaments in the abducted position, and a triangular shape to the rima glottidis. In Figure 6.4B, the arytenoids are abducted *and* rotated, the vocal ligaments are widely abducted, and the rima has a rhomboid shape. Not all authorities, however, agree that there is significant rotational movement at the cricoarytenoid joints. Movements at the cricoarytenoid joints are therefore used to vary the *size and shape* of the rima glottidis. The cricoarytenoid joints, however, also allow a certain amount of anteroposterior movement. When the arytenoids are pulled forwards they will relax the vocal ligaments. These movements are limited by the strong posterior ligaments of the joints. A backward pull on the arytenoids increases tension in the ligaments.

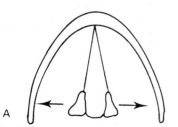
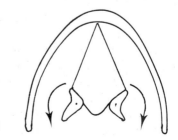

Fig. 6.4 View of the arytenoid cartilages from above. A: Sliding movement. B: Rotational movement.

2. The muscles of the larynx

The muscles which move the laryngeal cartilages at the cricothyroid and cricoarytenoid joints are called the 'intrinsic muscles of the larynx'. Extrinsic muscles pass between the larynx and neighbouring structures and move the larynx as a whole. The intrinsic muscles may be divided functionally into three groups: first, there are muscles which move the epiglottis and close the laryngeal inlet; secondly, there are muscles responsible for abduction and adduction of the cords; and finally, there are muscles which affect tension in the cords.

a. The inlet

Muscle fibres are found in each aryepiglottic fold extending from the apex of the arytenoid cartilage to the side of the epiglottis (Fig. 6.5A). The bundle is called the 'aryepiglottic muscle'. Fibres may be traced from the posterior end of each aryepiglottic muscle across the back of the larynx to the opposite arytenoid cartilage. These *oblique arytenoid* muscles form an 'X' at the back of the arytenoid cartilages. The aryepiglottic muscles and the oblique arytenoids form a sphincter at the inlet of the larynx. Their contraction brings the aryepiglottic folds together, and the arytenoid cartilages closer to the tubercle of the epiglottis. In addition to these, muscle fibres sweep up from the thyroid cartilage into the epiglottis on each side. These fibres constitute the thyroepiglottic muscles whose action is to open the inlet of the larynx (Fig. 6.5B).

b. Abduction and adduction of the cords

There is only one pair of abductors of the vocal cords, the *posterior cricoarytenoids*. Each arises from the back of the lamina of the cricoid and its fibres converge onto the lateral angle of the arytenoid cartilage, a point referred to as the 'muscular process'. The upper fibres of the muscle are horizontal, and the lowest fibres almost vertical. Between these two extremes the fibres of the muscle pass in varying degrees of obliquity from origin to insertion. The upper fibres act by rotating the arytenoid so that its vocal process turns laterally, a movement which abducts the vocal cord. The

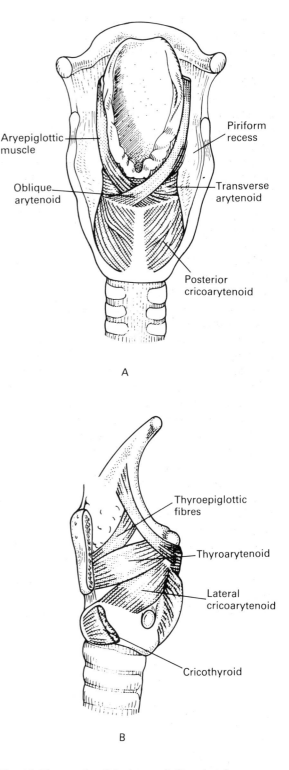

Fig. 6.5 The muscles of the larynx. A: Posterior view. B: Side view.

lower fibres of the muscle pull the arytenoid laterally with a gliding movement at the cricoarytenoid joint. The 'lateral cricoarytenoid' is the
principal adductor of the vocal cords. As its name
implies, it arises from the lateral side of the cricoid, and passes obliquely to the muscular process
of the arytenoid. It is assisted in bringing the arytenoids and vocal ligaments together by the *transverse arytenoid* muscle. This is composed of fibres
which pass horizontally from one arytenoid to the
other at the back of the larynx. The lateral cricoarytenoids close the glottis by rotating the arytenoid cartilages so that the vocal processes turn
medially, while the transverse arytenoid brings the
two arytenoids together by means of a gliding
movement at the cricoarytenoid joints. Figure 6.6
is a summary diagram of the muscle functions.

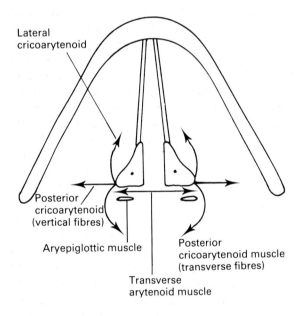

Fig. 6.6 Summary of the muscle actions

c. Tensors and relaxors

Alteration in tension of the vocal ligament is used
to alter the pitch of the voice, and is mainly controlled by the thyroarytenoid complex and the
cricothyroid. The *thyroarytenoid complex of muscle*
arises from the angle of the thyroid cartilage and
sweeps backwards to its insertion in the anterolateral surface of the arytenoid cartilage (Fig. 6.5B).

Some fibres, however, ascend as far as the epiglottis and are therefore known as the 'thyroepiglottic muscle'. This muscle widens the laryngeal
inlet and was therefore listed previously with the
muscles of the inlet. The main bulk of the thyroarytenoid complex draws the arytenoid cartilages
forwards and therefore relaxes the vocal ligament.
A deep, triangular bundle of fibres of the thyroarytenoid complex — the *vocalis* — lies parallel to
the vocal ligament. There is controversy concerning the origin and insertion of the fibres of this
bundle. It has been said that many arise from the
vocal ligament and pass back to the arytenoid.
Such fibres could selectively relax the posterior
part of the vocal ligament while the anterior part
remained tense. Some fibres of the vocalis arise
from the thyroid cartilage and insert into the cricovocal membrane below the vocal ligament. Contraction would pull up the membrane and create a
sharp edge to the vocal fold. Indeed, the cords
assume characteristic shapes and vibration patterns for each register. They are rounded and re-
laxed for chest tones, and sharp-edged for falsetto
tones. The vocalis fibres probably play a part in
producing these changes. The *cricothyroid* muscles
are intrinsic muscles which lie on the outer surface
of the larynx, and produce tension in the vocal
ligaments (see Fig. 8.3). The muscles are particularly involved in the production of the high tones
of the female voice. They act by tilting the cricoid
cartilage on the thyroid at the cricothyroid joints.
When the cricoid is fixed they produce a similar
effect by pulling the thyroid cartilage forwards.
The posterior cricoarytenoid muscles assist the
cricothyroids by pulling back on the arytenoids.
It will be seen from the foregoing account that
although we conveniently divide the muscles into
functional groups, muscles from one group often
act in harmony with muscles of another group,
and the division of labour is not clear-cut. Indeed,
even at dissection it is often difficult to define
where the fibres of one muscle end and those of an
adjacent muscle begin.

3. The interior of the larynx

Mucous membrane covers the cartilages, membranes and muscles of the larynx. As it is reflected
from the tongue onto the epiglottis, it forms one

median and two lateral glossoepiglottic folds. The depression on each side of the median fold is called the 'vallecula'. The membrane changes from a stratified squamous type to a ciliated columnar type at the back of the epiglottis, although areas of stratified squamous epithelium are found in places above the vocal cords. The inlet of the larynx may be traced from the epiglottis in front, around the aryepiglottic folds on either side to the mucous membrane stretching between the arytenoid cartilages at the back. The corniculate and cuneiform cartilages are found within each fold, where they present as two small tubercles (see Fig. 6.7). Between the outer and inner walls, the mucous membrane forms a piriform recess on either side (see Fig. 6.5A). Each recess is bounded in front by the thyrohyoid membrane and thyroid cartilage and posteromedially by the mucous membrane covering the aryepiglottic fold, thyroepiglottic muscle, and the saccule. It should be emphasised that the plane of the inlet of the larynx is almost vertical. It leads into the upper part of the larynx called the 'vestibule'. This part of the larynx extends from the inlet to the vestibular ligaments. Mucous membrane lines the vestibule and covers the ligaments to produce the vestibular folds. The gap between the two vestibular folds is called the 'rima vestibuli'. The middle of the larynx is the small area which extends from the level of the rima vestibuli to the rima glottidis. Mucous membrane balloons out between the vestibular and vocal ligaments as the sinus of the larynx. A narrow opening leads from the anterior aspect of this recess to a further cavity called the 'saccule of the larynx'. This pouch extends upwards on the outer side of the quadrangular membrane. Its mucous membrane contains many mucous glands. The outer surface of both sinus and saccule are clothed with the muscles at the side of the larynx, namely thyroarytenoid and thyroepiglottic muscles. Contraction of these muscles squeezes the saccule and sinus so expressing lubricating mucus onto the surface of the vocal fold. The middle part of the laryngeal cavity is the smallest part of the larynx, the rima glottidis being its narrowest section. The lower part of the laryngeal cavity extends from the vocal folds to the trachea. Mucous membrane is firmly adherent to the vocal ligaments, and is of stratified squamous type, which is well adapted to withstand frictional stress.

4. The nerve supply of the larynx

The nerve supply for the larynx comes from the vagus nerve through superior and recurrent laryngeal branches. The superior laryngeal nerve leaves the vagus high in the neck, and after passing deep to both carotids it divides into internal and external branches. The internal laryngeal nerve enters the larynx by piercing the thyrohyoid membrane and supplies sensation to the mucous membrane of the larynx above the vocal cords. Once through the thyrohyoid membrane, it lies beneath the mucous membrane of the piriform fossa, and supplies the fossa with sensation. In its upper part, the nerve supplies both surfaces of the epiglottis, the aryepiglottic fold, and the vallecula. Some taste buds are found on the posterior surface of the epiglottis and the taste pathway from them passes back in vagal fibres. The internal laryngeal nerve ends close to or within the substance of the inferior constrictor, where it unites with branches from the recurrent laryngeal nerve. The external laryngeal branch of the superior laryngeal nerve supplies the cricothyroid muscle. In its course towards this muscle on the outside of the larynx, it is closely associated with the superior thyroid artery, and must be protected during operations on the thyroid gland (see Ch. 8).

The recurrent laryngeal nerve enters the larynx behind the cricothyroid joint and inferior cornu of the thyroid cartilage. It supplies all of the intrinsic muscles of the larynx except the cricothyroid, and sensation to the mucous membrane below the vocal folds. Terminal branches anastomose with those of the superior laryngeal nerve. The cricopharyngeal part of the inferior constrictor is often supplied by twigs from either the recurrent nerve or the external laryngeal nerve. Occasionally the recurrent nerve divides before it enters the larynx, the separation sometimes being into sensory and motor bundles. Usually, however, there is no evidence of sorting of fibres in this way. During its course towards the larynx, the recurrent laryngeal nerve is closely associated with the inferior thyroid artery, and damage to the nerve must be avoided during thyroidectomy (see Ch. 8).

5. Injuries to the laryngeal nerves

Accounts of the results of laryngeal nerve injury in the literature are often confusing even though it would seem a straightforward pattern on theoretical grounds. This is especially so as far as recurrent laryngeal nerve injury is concerned. There are several reasons for this apparent confusion. Many lesions that have been described have occurred from accidental damage to a laryngeal nerve at the time of thyroid surgery. Others have been the result of a tumour in the neck or a tumour involving the left recurrent laryngeal nerve in the thorax. It is thus often impossible to be certain whether the nerve lesion has been complete, or if incomplete, which fibres have been involved. It has already been noted that the recurrent nerve often divides before entering the larynx, and therefore one or other bundle may be partially or completely divided. Postoperative oedema may also complicate the picture of nerve damage. Added to these uncertainties, anomalous nerve supply to the laryngeal muscles, and connections between the laryngeal nerves themselves may affect the clinical picture. The position and texture of the affected cord may change with the passage of time because of contraction of denervated muscle.

CASE 1

Phyllis Pulley, a 40-year-old housewife and active member of an amateur dramatic group, was admitted for thyroid surgery. After discharge from hospital, she complained that her voice was husky, easily fatigued, and lower pitched than before the operation. This prevented her participation in plays by the drama group. Laryngoscopy revealed that the right vocal cord was irregular and at a lower level than the left cord. It bulged on expiration. Apart from this, the cords abducted and adducted normally. It was assumed that the recurrent laryngeal nerves were normal, but that the right external laryngeal nerve had been damaged. Phyllis was referred to a speech therapist for rehabilitation of the voice. Considerable improvement was achieved during the following 3 months, but she was left with permanent weakness of the voice. The effects of damage to the external laryngeal nerve should not be underestimated; they can cause troublesome problems.

On theoretical grounds it would be logical to assume that injury to the recurrent laryngeal nerve would result in paralysis of all the intrinsic muscles on the side of the lesion except the cricothyroid. The vocal cord should therefore be near its adducted position and should be tense because of the unopposed action of the cricothyroid. There should be sensory loss below the vocal cords. Laryngoscopic examination, however, may show the affected cord to be abducted or adducted. It may also be in an intermediate position, but it must be admitted that it is often difficult to estimate any exact position between full abduction and adduction at laryngoscopic examination. The term 'cadaveric' position has been used to describe an abducted cord, but a 'cadaveric' position implies that all the laryngeal muscles are paralysed and it should therefore be used when there is a complete vagal lesion. 'Cadaveric' also implies that rigor mortis exists. It is probably best dropped from the laryngeal vocabulary and descriptive adjectives limited to 'abducted', 'adducted', 'fixed', 'mobile', 'straight' and 'bowed'. Injury to one recurrent laryngeal nerve may thus result in the affected cord being fixed in an adducted position or in an abducted position. Indeed, with the lapse of time an abducted cord may gradually adduct. If the cord is fixed in the adducted position the subject will complain of dyspnoea on exertion. If the cord is abducted the complaint will be of hoarseness and weakness of the voice without dyspnoea. It has been stated that trauma which partially injures the recurrent laryngeal nerve results in more damage to the abductor than to the adductor innervation. This has been referred to as 'Simon's law'. Partial damage may well account for the variability of position of the cord in recurrent laryngeal nerve damage. As time goes by, the opposite vocal cord adapts its position, and there is often some improvement. Unilateral damage to the recurrent laryngeal nerve, which causes hoarseness, resolves completely in half of the patients. Bilateral paralysis of the recurrent laryngeal nerves, which results in adducted cords, causes both dyspnoea and hoarseness. Bilateral palsy causes early complete loss of the voice, but half of the patients recover some voice.

If damage to a recurrent nerve is noticed at operation, an attempt can be made to establish an end-to-end anastomosis. Results, however, are not always good. If the final result of a recurrent nerve lesion is a fixed abducted cord, the main complaint is of weakness of the voice. If recovery does not occur, techniques to improve the quality and strength of the voice are available. The arytenoid and affected cord may be repositioned more medially and fixed to the cricoid. Another method of bringing the vocal cord closer to the midline involves the injection of teflon just lateral to the vocal cord, and this pushes the affected cord towards the midline. Alternatively, strips of cartilage may be implanted into the paraglottic space, to push the cord closer to the midline. Bilateral vocal cord adduction is a greater problem, but techniques have been devised to implant nerve muscle preparations of the ansa cervicalis and segments of strap muscle into the posterior cricoarytenoid muscle. If this operation is successful it establishes a laryngeal abductor once again. Such an operation, however, calls for a great deal of technical skill. A simpler form of treatment is to ablate part of one vocal cord with a carbon dioxide laser. This simple technique produces an adequate airway.

CASE 2

Jimmy Jolly, a 12-year-old schoolboy, suffered from a sarcoma of the occipital bone. This had infiltrated the jugular foramen and had caused damage to the 9th, 10th and 11th cranial nerves. He had received radiotherapy for the tumour, which had regressed. The cranial nerve lesions, however, resulted in derangement of the normal protective function of the larynx, with the result that he had laryngeal incompetence. When he tried to swallow, fluid entered the larynx, and precipitated a bout of explosive coughing. Saliva accumulated in the mouth, and was occasionally aspirated.

Normal swallowing takes place by a series of reflexes which are coordinated by the deglutition centre in the medulla. Reflex activity follows stimulation of the mechanoreceptors of the mouth and pharyngeal wall. Afferent impulses pass in the trigeminal nerve, the glossopharyngeal nerve, and the pharyngeal and internal laryngeal branches of the vagus. These impulses pass bilaterally to the brain-stem centre. Efferent impulses leave the brain from the trigeminal, glossopharyngeal, vagal and hypoglossal nuclei. Most of the fibres which reach the larynx and pharynx, however, originate in the nucleus ambiguus. Cortical representation is bilateral, with partial decussation of the fibres

before reaching the nucleus ambiguus. This means that only bilateral cortical lesions will cause upper motor neurone dysfunction of the larynx. Reflex activity results in elevation of the larynx and pharynx, and closure of the nasopharynx and laryngeal inlet. In addition, relaxation of the cricopharyngeal sphincter occurs and a peristaltic wave of contraction passes from the pharynx down the oesophagus.

Jimmy was suffering from combined motor and sensory deficits of the pathways involved in deglutition. In order to make life more comfortable, and prevent aspiration, an epiglottopexy was performed. The epiglottis was fixed to the aryepiglottic folds, a small opening being left in the posterior part of the inlet to preserve phonation and an airway.

6. Laryngoscopic examination

The inlet of the larynx may be examined by means of an angled mirror passed over the back of the tongue into the oral part of the pharynx. In order to do this, the examiner grasps the tongue with a gauze swab and pulls it forwards (Fig. 6.7). The oral part of the pharynx is lightly sprayed with local anaesthetic. The mirror is warmed over a flame before insertion, to prevent misting of its surface by the patient's breath. The epiglottis and its tubercle will be seen in the mirror, and the aryepiglottic folds can be identified on either side. The piriform fossae should be inspected on either side of the inlet. Inside the larynx, both vestibular and vocal folds should be visible. The vocal folds are pearly white in colour because of the strong attachment of the mucous membrane to the ligament and the lack of a submucous layer of blood vessels. If the patient is asked to make a sound, movement of the vocal cords should be observed.

CASE 3

Roland Rumball, a 45-year-old, 20 stone antique dealer, felt a fish bone stick in his throat while eating a trout. When seen in the emergency unit, an indirect laryngoscopy was attempted without success. A lateral radiograph of the neck did not reveal a fish bone, and so he was told that there was no fish bone in the throat, and sent home. 24 hours later, however, Roland returned to the emergency unit with surgical emphysema (air in the subcutaneous tissues), and difficulty in breathing. Figure 6.8 is a soft tissue radiograph or

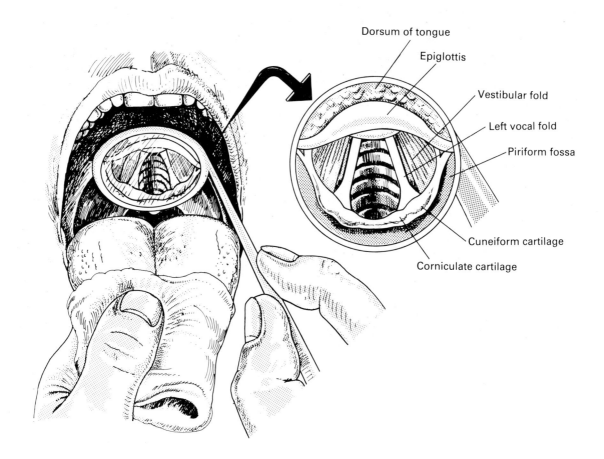

Fig. 6.7 Indirect laryngoscopy

'xerogram', and shows widespread surgical emphysema in Roland's neck. The fishbone was still not visible radiologically. The student should remember that only about 75% of bones are visible radiologically at soft tissue exposures. Trout and mackerel have poorly calcified bones, while salmon bones are more opaque. Indirect laryngoscopy is the best way of detecting a bone. Roland was admitted to hospital, and at laryngoscopy a large fish bone was removed from the right piriform fossa, where it had pierced the thyrohyoid membrane. Roland made a good recovery, and decided to start a reducing diet.

The larynx may be examined by direct laryngoscopy with a laryngoscope. This technique is used during induction of anaesthesia for tracheal intubation. It is also used during intubation to cs-

tablish an emergency airway in certain unconscious patients. Tracheal intubation is also occasionally performed in the conscious patient when there is inadequate spontaneous clearing of the tracheobronchial tree. Laryngoscopes come in several sizes, for use in the adult, the child and the infant. The handle contains a battery, and the light is concealed in the blade. Laryngoscope blades may be curved or straight. The curved blade is designed to indirectly lift the epiglottis off the larynx (Fig. 6.9A). Its tip is placed above the epiglottis at the base of the tongue, and by pulling on the glossoepiglottic fold, the epiglottis is lifted. The curved blade, therefore, does not touch the larynx itself. It produces less trauma and less reflex stimulation of the larynx than the straight blade. The straight blade, on the other hand, is designed to pick up the epiglottis directly (Fig. 6.9B).

Every medical student should learn how to use a laryngoscope. With the mouth held open, the patient's neck is extended with the chin thrust forwards. The laryngoscope is held firmly with the left hand, and the blade inserted through the right corner of the mouth. The tongue is pushed to the left side of the mouth so that it does not obscure the view along the blade. The lips and teeth should be protected from injury during the procedure. The laryngoscope blade is moved to the sagittal plane, and the blade passed over the back of the tongue until the epiglottis comes into view. While this procedure is taking place, the other hand should be moved to the patient's occiput to hold the head tilted backward. After seeing the epiglottis, the arytenoids will come into view in the midline. Finally, the vocal cords will be seen by pulling the handle upwards at right angles to the blade (arrow in Fig. 6.9A). When carrying out this latter procedure, the teeth should not be used as a fulcrum. If the view is not sufficient, a helper can assist by pushing the larynx backward. This often

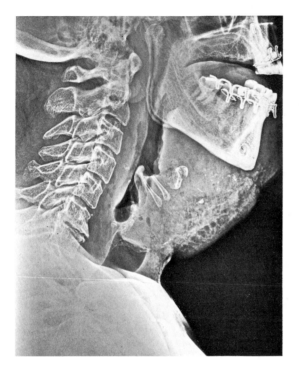

Fig. 6.8 Roland Rumball. Xerogram of the neck.

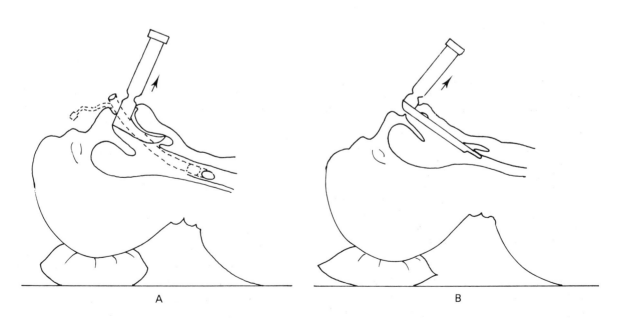

A

B

Fig. 6.9 A: The curved laryngoscope. B: The straight laryngoscope.

brings the cords into view. When intubating small children, the student must remember that the larynx is located relatively higher than in the adult. The epiglottis is U-shaped, and the larynx funnel-shaped, with its narrowest diameter at the level of the cricoid. During endoctracheal intubation, the tube is passed along the blade, into the larynx between the cords, and finally into the trachea. The cuff around the distal end of the tube is inflated. This comfortably fixes the distal end of the tube in the trachea (Fig. 6.9A). At the start of extubation, the cuff is deflated, and the mouth and oropharynx suctioned before the tube is removed.

The larynx is occasionally obstructed by a foreign body. This is particularly prone to happen in a subject partially intoxicated, who is eating and talking at the same time. It is thus seen from time to time in restaurants. The obstructing bolus is usually an inadequately chewed portion of meat. The subject clasps his throat, and soon becomes cyanosed. Eventually he loses consciousness. When confronted by such a problem, it is important to differentiate between an obstructed larynx and a heart attack. When first seen, the patient must be asked if he can talk. If this is possible, then clearly there is no laryngeal obstruction. In order to expel a bolus of food, the examiner stands behind the patient and clasps his chest in an embrace. The fists lie in front over the patient's lower sternum. The patient is bent forwards, and several sharp constrictive movements are applied to the chest. If this does not succeed in removing the bolus, the back of the patient is struck several times, and the manoeuvre repeated. Very rarely, it may be possible to remove the bolus by using two fingers placed down the subject's throat. In fact, some restaurants keep long curved forceps for this type of removal. Very rarely, it will be necessary to make an artificial airway below the vocal cords. The simplest way of doing this in an emergency is by a cricothyroid membrane puncture. The larynx is grasped between the thumb and finger, and a stab incision is made through the cricothyroid membrane. The danger with this procedure is damage to the vocal cords, and laryngeal stenosis after healing. At other times, a formal tracheostomy and insertion of a tube is required. There are many indications for such a procedure, ranging from an obstruction of

the larynx to problems such as multiple rib fractures in the chest. In this latter condition, ventilation may be inadequate, and a tube is inserted so that the patient may be ventilated mechanically. Although many conditions which require assisted ventilation can be controlled by an endotracheal tube at first, this will have to be replaced by a tracheostomy tube after a few days. The endotracheal tube cannot be left in place for longer than this, because it will ulcerate the interior of the larynx. To perform a tracheostomy, a transverse incision is made in the lower part of the neck. It is taken through skin and platysma and exposes the infrahyoid strap muscles. The midline between these muscles is opened, and the isthmus of the thyroid gland exposed. This is clamped and incised. A window is made in the trachea, usually in the shape of an inverted U. The edge of this tracheal flap can be sutured to the lower edge of the wound. This helps to direct the tube into the tracheal cavity. Figure 6.10 shows a xerogram of a patient with a tracheostomy and the tube in place.

7. Radiology of the larynx

On a lateral view of the neck, the epiglottis is usually outlined by air in the pharynx. The cartilages of the larynx and the hyoid contain irregular speckles of calcification. It is important on such a radiograph not to confine the examination to the larynx. The cervical vertebral column and the prevertebral tissues must also be examined. Figure 6.11 is a tomogram of the larynx. The piriform fossae are seen on either side of the supraglottic region of the larynx. Both vestibular and vocal folds are seen, and the wide infraglottic compartment leading to the trachea is found below the vocal cords. CT scans of the larynx show great detail, and are especially useful in showing the extent of tumour involvement. At such examinations, the thyroid density may be increased by intravenous contrast medium. This can also be used to show the internal carotid artery and internal jugular vein.

8. Lymphatic drainage

The lymphatics of the larynx form two distinct systems, one above and the other below the vocal

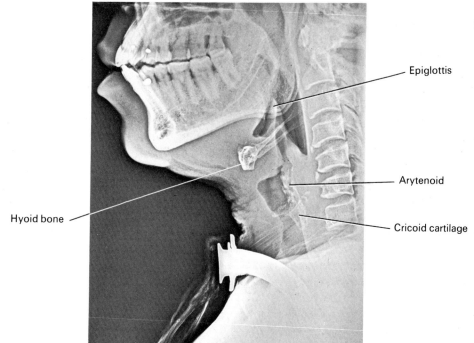

Fig. 6.10 Xerogram of a subject with a tracheostomy

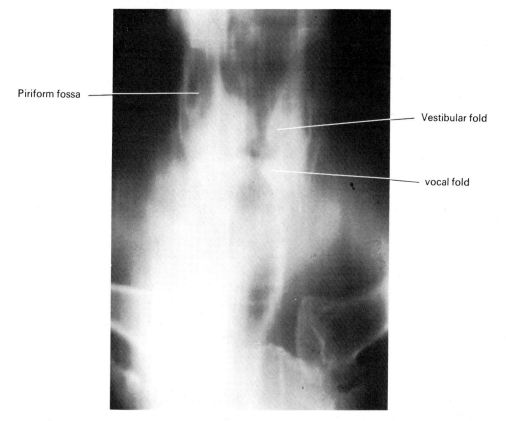

Fig. 6.11 Tomogram of the larynx

cords. Anastomoses between the two systems occur in the posterior wall of the larynx. The lymphatics from the upper group pierce the thyrohyoid membrane and follow the superior laryngeal vessels. They reach the upper deep cervical nodes. The lower vessels pierce the cricovocal membrane and drain into pretracheal nodes on the cricovocal membrane, and paratracheal nodes along the course of the recurrent laryngeal nerve. Efferents from these nodes drain into the lower deep cervical nodes. Some lymphatics from the lower part of the larynx pierce the membrane between the cricoid and first tracheal ring and drain into the lower deep cervical nodes. Lymphatics from the trachea drain into pretracheal, paratracheal and deep cervical nodes.

The anatomical description of the muscles of the larynx and movement of the vocal folds in this chapter represents the 'classical' view of function. Many new techniques have been developed by scientists concerned with speech to study such function in more detail. It is becoming clear that the movements of the folds, and their alteration in shape, are more complicated than suggested by the 'classical' description. Indeed, some assumptions of muscle action may be quite wrong. One technique used to study vocal cord movement involves taking 'flash' radiographs of the functioning larynx. A series of four consecutive flash pictures is shown in Figure 6.12.

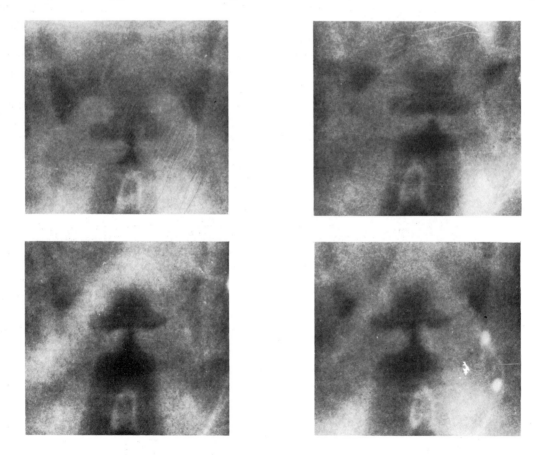

Fig. 6.12 Flash sequence of larynx taken at 30 μs. X-ray pulses, 280 KV. Sequence shows progression of movement of normally vibrating vocal cords during the production of a sustained [a] vowel at the male adult speaker's modal frequency of 124 Hz. (By kind permission of Professor A. J. Fourcin, Department of Phonetics and Linguistics, University College London, and Professor R. J. Berry and Mr N. J. Nascoe, Department of Oncology and Nuclear Medicine, Middlesex Hospital Medical School.) A: Vocal folds immediately prior to complete closure. B: Vocal folds at maximum point of contact. C: Vocal folds abducted, at 20% of larynx period interval between closure points. D: Abduction at 60% of the larynx period interval. The folds are taking up the shape seen in 'A' prior to closure.

7

THE PHARYNX

The pharynx is a large muscular tube located behind the nose, mouth, and larynx. It extends from the base of the skull to the lower border of the cricoid cartilage where it is continuous with the oesophagus. This lower limit is set at the level of the 6th cervical vertebra.

1. Muscles of the pharynx

Most of the muscles of the pharynx are arranged horizontally as the superior, middle and inferior constrictors. There are, in addition, three longitudinally arranged muscles, the stylopharyngeus, the salpingopharyngeus and the palatopharyngeus (Figs. 7.1, 7.2). The *superior constrictor* arises in front from the medial pterygoid plate and its pterygoid hamulus, and the mylohyoid line on the inner surface of the mandible. Between these bony origins the fibres interdigitate with those of the buccinator at a pterygomandibular raphe. A few

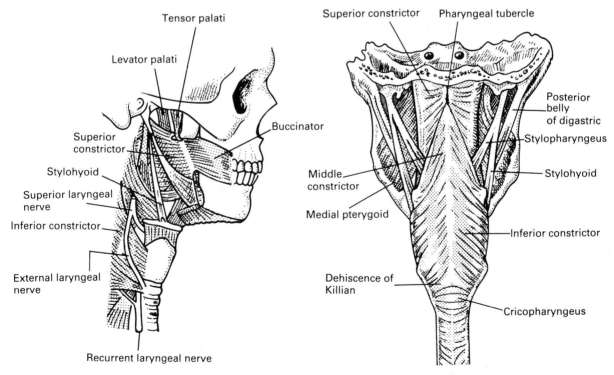

Fig. 7.1 The pharynx

Fig. 7.2 A posterior view of the pharynx

fibres of the constrictor also arise from the side of the tongue. Traced around the pharynx, the fibres end in a median raphe with the fibres of the constrictor of the opposite side. The upper fibres reach the pharyngeal tubercle on the occipital bone. The upper border of the superior constrictor is free, so that there is a triangular interval between it, the base of the skull and the upper part of the medial pterygoid plate. The auditory tube passes through the front of this gap next to the medial pterygoid plate, and the plate is scalloped to receive the pharyngeal end of the tube. The rest of the interval is closed by pharyngobasilar fascia. The auditory tube is closely related to two palatine muscles which arise from the base of the skull, the tensor veli palatini on the outside of the pharynx and the levator veli palatini on the inside. Indeed, both these muscles partially arise from the cartilage of the auditory tube. A band of muscle arises from the upper surface of the palatine aponeurosis, and passes around the pharynx on the inner surface of the superior constrictor. These fibres have been described by Passavant and by Whillis. The band is called the 'palatopharyngeal sphincter' or Passavant's muscle. During deglutition, the palate is raised, and simultaneously the palatopharyngeal sphincter produces a ridge on the posterior pharyngeal wall. Apposition of the palate and ridge closes off the nasal part of the pharynx. The sphincter is hypertrophied in babies with complete cleft palate. Not all agree that there is such a definitive layer of muscle under normal circumstances, and it has been suggested that the ridge is simply a fold of mucous membrane produced when the longitudinal muscle of the pharynx contracts.

The *middle constrictor* is fan-shaped, and arises from the lesser cornu of the hyoid, the stylohyoid ligament, and the greater cornu of the hyoid bone. The fibres insert into the median raphe at the back of the pharynx, the upper fibres overlapping the superior constrictor and the lower fibres passing deep to the inferior constrictor. The *inferior constrictor* arises from both the thyroid and cricoid cartilages. It is thus said to be composed of thyropharyngeal and cricopharyngeal parts. The muscle arises from the oblique line of the thyroid cartilage and from a band of fibrous tissue which stretches from the line to the cricoid cartilage, and bridges

across the cricothyroid muscle. These fibres insert posteriorly into the median fibrous raphe. The cricopharyngeal part of the inferior constrictor arises from the cricoid cartilage. Its fibres form a complete sphincter, and are continuous below with the muscular fibres of the oesophagus. Apart from the appendix, the junction between the inferior constrictor and the oesophagus is the narrowest part of the alimentary canal.

CASE 1

Sir William Wipp, a 40-year-old country estate owner, had noticed difficulty in swallowing (dysphagia) for a number of years. In recent months this had become so bad that he was only able to take very small meals. If he attempted to eat more, he regurgitated undigested food. Food also tended to enter the larynx and cause a fit of coughing.

Dysphagia is a common presenting symptom in patients with pharyngeal and oesophageal problems. Patients are remarkably accurate at siting oesophageal obstruction, and should therefore be asked to point to the level of the obstruction. As part of the investigation of the dysphagia, Sir William had a barium swallow (Fig. 7.3). This showed a pharyngeal pouch or diverticulum at the lower pharynx. The usual place for a such a protrusion is through the back of the pharynx, just above the cricopharyngeus. Here, the posterior wall of the pharynx is relatively weak and has been called the 'dehiscence of Killian'. Killian made a careful study of this part of the pharyngeal wall, and found the wall to be deficient in muscular strength. An increase in the intrapharyngeal pressure will start a herniation of mucous membrane, and failure of relaxation of cricopharyngeus adds to the problem. Such a pharyngeal diverticulum, although usually midline in position, protrudes to one or other side of the pharynx, and may present as a swelling at the side of the neck. In its early stages the pouch causes a feeling of a 'lump' in the throat, but soon dysphagia is evident. When the pouch fills with food during a meal, it overflows into the pharynx.

Operation notes
The diverticulum is not always easy to identify at operation, therefore an oesophagoscope was passed and the diverticulum packed with gauze. The pharynx was approached through an incision placed over the lower anterior border of the sternocleidomastoid. The approach is usually through

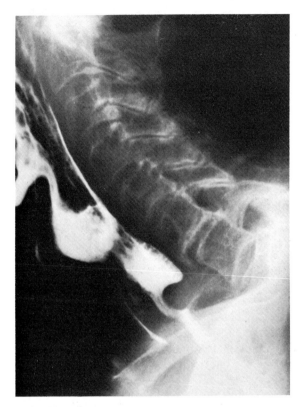

Fig. 7.3 Sir William Wipp. Barium swallow.

the left side of the neck, because the oesophagus passes to the left of the vertebral bodies. The muscle was retracted backward and the omohyoid muscle exposed, and transected. The thyroid gland was retracted towards the midline and the carotid sheath retracted backward. The inferior thyroid artery, which often crosses over the diverticulum, was located and ligated. The recurrent laryngeal nerve was identified in the tracheo-oesophageal groove. The diverticulum was closely bound to the oesophagus by enveloping fibres of the cricopharyngeus. These were separated from the sac, and the diverticulum exposed. The neck of the sac was opened and a finger inserted. The cricopharyngeal muscle fibres were made prominent over the finger and cut (cricopharyngeal myotomy). The neck of the sac was transfixed and the diverticulum excised. Sir William made a good recovery and was soon enjoying good food again at his country house.

The cricopharyngeal muscle was first described by Valsalva in 1717. It forms a sphincter at the upper end of the oesophagus, which is normally closed. Dysphagia associated with hypochromic microcytic anaemia, angular stomatitis, glossitis and koilonychia, is not uncommon. The group of conditions is called the Paterson-Brown Kelly syndrome in the UK and the Plummer-Vinson syndrome in the USA. Some of these patients, who are usually female, present with a postcricoid web. This curious condition is sometimes seen as a definite diaphragm at oesophagoscopy, but at other times is only seen radiologically. A very small number of patients with the syndrome develop postcricoid carcinoma.

The *stylopharyngeus* is a slender muscle which arises from the medial side of the styloid process. It enters the pharynx between the superior and middle constrictors and some of its fibres merge with those of the pharyngeal constrictor. Others insert into the posterior border of the thyroid cartilage. It is accompanied by the glossopharyngeal nerve, which winds around the posterior border and lateral side of the muscle to gain the gap between the constrictors. The *palatopharyngeus* arises by two fasciculi from the upper surface of the palatine aponeurosis. The anterior fasciculus, the larger of the two, arises in front of the insertion of the levator veli palatini. The posterior fasciculus arises behind this insertion. The muscle descends to insert into the posterior border of the thyroid cartilage, and the pharyngeal wall. In so doing it raises a prominent palatopharyngeal fold behind the palatine tonsil. The *salpingopharyngeus* is a small muscle which arises from the lower part of the auditory tube cartilage. The fibres blend with those of the palatopharyngeus.

2. The interior of the pharynx

Internally the pharynx may be divided into nasal, oral and laryngeal parts. The *nasal part of the pharynx* lies behind the nose, and communicates with it through the posterior apertures of the nose. The roof of the nasal part of the pharynx consists of the sphenoid and occipital bones, and the anterior arch of the atlas. The auditory tube opens into the lateral wall of the nasal pharynx about 1 cm behind the posterior end of the inferior nasal concha. The cartilaginous end of the tube produces a tubal elevation above and behind the opening, and the salpingopharyngeus raises a fold of mucous membrane as it descends from the tube. Behind the tubal elevation is the pharyngeal recess of Rosenmüller at the junction of the lateral and posterior pharyngeal walls. A collection of lymphoid tissue called the 'pharyngeal tonsil' lies in the mucous membrane of the roof and posterior wall of the nasal part of the pharynx. Some of this tissue extends as far laterally as the auditory tube, where it is called the 'tubal tonsil'. The pharyngeal tonsil, present at birth, increases in size during the first 6 years of life. During late childhood, the pharyngeal tonsil often atrophies and very little can be seen in most adults. It occasionally enlarges in childhood, and obstructs the nasopharynx. These so-called 'adenoids' will then need to be removed surgically. A small midline recess called the 'pharyngeal bursa', may be found in the centre of the pharyngeal tonsil. During development, the notochord lies within the basilar part of the occipital bone close to the pharynx, and is in fact attached to the endodermal lining of the primitive pharynx. With the growth of the base of the skull and the notochord, this attachment pulls out a small diverticulum called the 'pouch of Luschka'. The pharyngeal bursa is thought to be a remnant of this pouch. A Tornwaldt's cyst may occur in the region of the pharyngeal bursa, and this is also thought to have an embryological origin. A pharyngeal hypophysis is sometimes seen as a small dimple at a higher level than the pharyngeal bursa. It is possibly a remnant of Rathke's pouch, but this is by no means certain. When present, it is submucous or periosteal in position. The opening of the nasopharynx into the oral part of the pharynx is called the 'pharyngeal isthmus', and must be closed during the act of swallowing. This is achieved by elevation of the soft palate and contraction of the palatopharyngeal sphincter.

The *oral part of the pharynx* is located behind the mouth, and communicates with it through the oropharyngeal isthmus. On each side the isthmus is formed by the palatoglossal fold or arch, formed by the underlying palatoglossus. The palatopharyngeus raises a ridge behind the palatoglossus, the two folds being separated by the tonsillar sinus. Both folds can usually be seen in the mouth, and are often referred to as the 'anterior and posterior pillars of the fauces' or the 'palatoglossal and palatopharyngeal arches'. The

palatine tonsil lies in the sinus between the folds. The palatine tonsils are present at birth; they enlarge during childhood, but usually diminish in size from the age of puberty. The free surface of the tonsil is excavated by deep tonsillar crypts which penetrate deep into the tonsillar substance. At the upper pole of the tonsil is a large, horizontally placed, intratonsillar cleft. This has been called the 'supratonsillar fossa', but the term is somewhat inaccurate, as the cleft is found within tonsillar tissue and not above it. Very occasionally a fold of mucous membrane may be found extending backward from the lower part of the palatoglossal fold to the tongue. This is a remnant of a fold found during development of the tonsil in fetal life.

On a deeper plane, the tonsil extends upwards into the palate and downwards into the dorsum of the tongue. Its lateral surface is covered by a layer of fibrous tissue, called the 'capsule', which separates it from the tonsillar bed. The bed is muscular and formed by the superior constrictor of the pharynx. The styloglossus, and the ascending palatine branch of the facial artery are located immediately outside the tonsillar bed. Indeed, the facial artery itself is often closely related to the superior constrictor in this region. The glossopharyngeal nerve is also close to the outer surface of the bed, and a transient 9th nerve palsy occasionally occurs as a result of postoperative oedema after tonsillectomy. The internal carotid artery and the ascending pharyngeal artery lie vertically on the outer surface of the constrictor behind the tonsillar bed. The tonsil is supplied with blood by the *tonsillar branch of the facial artery*. This vessel, accompanied by venae comitantes, pierces the superior constrictor in the lower part of the tonsillar sinus. Twigs from the *ascending palatine branch of the facial artery* also pierce the superior constrictor to reach the tonsil, and branches from the *lingual artery* enter the lower pole of the tonsil. The *ascending pharyngeal branch of the external carotid* also gives twigs to the palatine tonsil, the branch entering the palate in company with the levator palati. Blood also reaches the tonsil by means of the *greater palatine branch of the maxillary artery*. One or two veins pierce the superior constrictor in the lower part of the tonsillar sinus and usually drain into the facial vein. Often, one of the palatine veins is particularly large. It is called the 'paratonsillar vein' because it descends from the palate across the capsule of the tonsil where it pierces the superior constrictor. During tonsillectomy this vein may be injured and cause troublesome bleeding from the upper part of the tonsillar sinus.

The *laryngeal part of the pharynx* extends to the level of the cricoid cartilage. In front is the inlet of the larynx and the posterior aspects of the arytenoid and cricoid cartilages. The details of the inlet are given in Chapter 6.

3. Nerve supply to the pharynx

The sensory nerve supply from the nasal part of the pharynx is transmitted through a pharyngeal branch of the pterygopalatine ganglion. This reaches the ganglion from the pharynx through the palatinovaginal canal, and the fibres continue to the maxillary nerve. Their cell bodies lie in the trigeminal ganglion. The main sensory nerve supply to the oral part of the pharynx, including most of the surface of the palatine tonsil, comes from the glossopharyngeal nerve. Some of the mucous membrane over the tonsil is, however, supplied by branches from the lesser palatine nerve. Pain from tonsillitis is often referred to the ear, through the tympanic branch of the glossopharyngeal nerve. Sensation to the mucous membrane of the laryngeal part of the pharynx is supplied by laryngeal nerves (see Ch. 6). The motor nerve supply to the constrictor muscles of the pharynx comes from the pharyngeal plexus. The motor input into this plexus is the pharyngeal branch of the vagus nerve. This carries cranial accessory fibres to innervate the constrictors, palatopharyngeus and salpingopharyngeus. Stylopharyngeus has a separate nerve supply from the glossopharyngeal nerve. Postganglionic sympathetic fibres enter into the plexus from the superior cervical sympathetic ganglion, and parasympathetic fibres reach the plexus through the glossopharyngeal nerve. Glossopharyngeal sensory fibres from the oral part of the pharynx also pass through the plexus.

4. The fascial spaces around the pharynx

A fascial space exists behind the pharynx between it and the prevertebral muscles and fascia. This retropharyngeal space is important clinically because it can become infected. In childhood, such an infection may result from lymph node involvement secondary to an upper respiratory tract infection. The child presents with a high temperature. The swelling, which appears on one side of the posterior pharyngeal wall, may obstruct the airway. Prevertebral and retropharyngeal abscesses in the adult are usually secondary to tuberculous disease of the cervical vertebral column. When examining a radiograph of the neck, it is important not to omit an inspection of the cervical column and the prevertebral tissues. Figure 7.4 shows disease of the cervical spine. This patient has ankylosing spondylitis, and the anterior longitudinal ligament is ossified. The spine takes the appearance of a bamboo rod. The prevertebral soft tissue density is clearly seen in the upper part of this picture. It is normally narrow superiorly, but widens just above the level of the cricoid cartilage. The radiograph in Figure

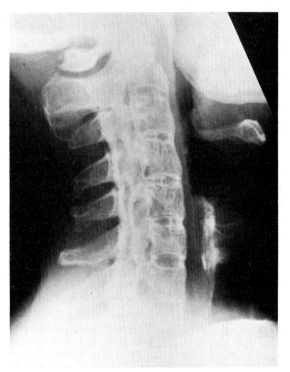

Fig. 7.4 Lateral radiograph of the neck of a subject with ankylosing spondylitis

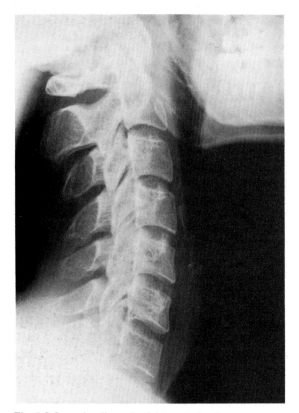

Fig. 7.5 Lateral radiograph of the neck showing a prevertebral swelling

7.5 is from a patient with a retropharyngeal infection from a small fish bone, which had perforated the back of the pharynx.

CASE 2

Petunia Poll was admitted to hospital for investigation of hoarseness. In order to leave the larynx free for inspection during laryngoscopy, the anaesthetist elected to pass a cannula directly into the trachea, and give the anaesthetic gases by this route. Following induction, the cannula was passed into the trachea and the anaesthetic machine started. With the first jet, the anaesthetist inspected the chest to make sure that the gases were filling the lungs. The chest did not rise, and he heard no gas movement with the stethoscope. A second jet was not given, the cannula was removed, and anaesthesia was continued by means of an endotracheal tube. The examination was unsuccessful, but while inspecting the larynx,

the surgeon noted that the back of the pharynx was bruised. Postoperatively, Petunia complained of pharyngeal discomfort and dysphagia. She was told of the initial difficulty, and advised to stay in hospital. Within 12 hours she had a pyrexia. A lateral radiograph of the neck showed a prevertebral swelling in front of the 5th, 6th and 7th cervical vertebrae (Fig. 7.6). It was assumed that the anaesthetist's needle had perforated the trachea and oesophagus, and entered the retropharyngeal and prevertebral tissues. Large doses of antibiotics were given, and the swelling subsided. She was left with no permanent side-effects, but decided to take legal action against the hospital. She did not win her case. The court ruled that the anaesthetist had acted correctly by recognising that the needle was not correctly placed, and by reverting to another form of anaesthesia.

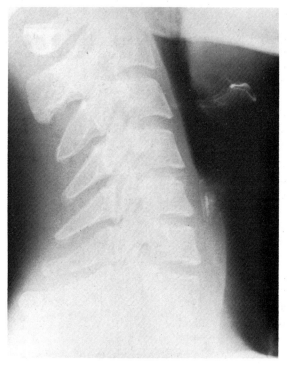

Fig. 7.6 Petunia Poll. Lateral radiograph of the neck.

CASE 3

Buddy Bradley, a 45-year-old mechanic at an oil rig, had a habit of holding objects in his mouth at work. While doing this one day, he accidentally swallowed a short piece of wire. This caused little immediate discomfort, and he went on working. By the following day, however, he had an uncomfortable feeling in the pharynx and had dysphagia. A lateral radiograph of the neck showed a small piece of wire lying behind the pharynx in front of the 5th and 6th cervical vertebrae within a soft tissue swelling (Fig. 7.7). At oesophagoscopy the end of the wire was found sticking through the posterior pharyngeal wall, and it proved an easy matter to remove the object. The swelling subsided with a course of antibiotics.

The retropharyngeal space connects laterally with a parapharyngeal space. This is bounded laterally by the pterygoid muscles, the mandible and the deep edge of the parotid gland. The medial boundary is the superior constrictor of the pharynx. The space extends from the base of the skull to the hyoid bone, where it is limited by the fascial covering of the submandibular gland. The space contains the carotid artery, the internal jugular vein, the vagus nerve, the sympathetic trunk, and the upper deep cervical lymph nodes. Infection in this space is rare, but when seen usually follows as a complication of tonsillitis. It may, however, on rare occasions be produced by an infection around the root of the lower 3rd molar tooth. Mastoid infection can also extend into the parapharyngeal space along the sheath of the digastric muscle. Infection in the air cells of the apex of the petrous temporal bone can also extend into the space.

If surgical drainage is required for a retropharyngeal abscess, the incision is placed over the posterior border of the sternocleidomastoid. The abscess is located by opening between the carotid sheath and the prevertebral muscles. The parapharyngeal space is approached by an incision along the anterior border of the sternocleidomastoid. A search is made between the muscle and the carotid sheath.

The pharynx may be outlined on a CT scan. Figure 7.8 is a tracing of some of the structures found on a CT scan through the nasopharynx. The auditory tube is usually outlined with air, as is the fossa of Rosenmüller behind it. The parapharyngeal space lies outside the nasopharynx, between it and the lateral pterygoid muscle. It contains the styloid process, the internal carotid artery and the internal jugular vein. The vessels may be outlined by intravenous contrast medium. The parotid fascia is of greater density than the subcutaneous

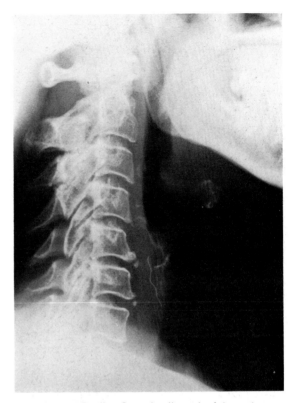

Fig. 7.7 Buddy Bradley. Lateral radiograph of the neck.

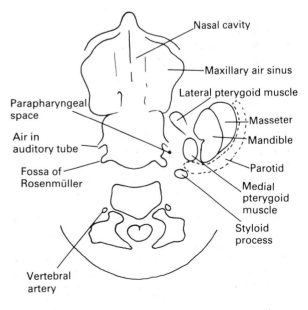

Fig. 7.8 Outline of a CT scan at the level of the nasopharynx

fat, and is therefore outlined. Intravenous contrast medium, which is taken up by the salivary gland, will increase the density of the parotid shadow.

5. Lymphatic drainage of the pharynx

Lymphatics from the pharynx pass directly to the deep cervical nodes, or indirectly through retro-pharyngeal or paratracheal nodes. The retropharyngeal lymph nodes lie behind the pharynx, in front of the prevertebral fascia, and consist of longitudinally arranged median and two lateral groups. Their efferents pass to the upper deep cervical lymph nodes. Lymph from the epiglottis runs to the infrahyoid nodes. Lymph vessels from the tonsil pierce the buccopharyngeal fascia and the superior constrictor muscle to reach the angle between the stylohyoid and the internal jugular vein. They enter the upper deep cervical lymph nodes, most of them ending in the jugulodigastric nodes.

6. Development of the pharynx

The developing pharynx gives a characteristic appearance to the early embryo. Pharyngeal or branchial arches are first visible between the fourth and fifth weeks of development, each arch being separated from its neighbour by a thin membrane of ectoderm and endoderm. On the outside of the embryo these ectodermal slits are called 'branchial clefts', while inside the pharynx, endodermal branchial pouches lie between the arches. Developmental abnormalities in the region give rise to problems associated with the face, palate, pharynx, thyroid and parathyroid glands.

The 1st branchial arch forms maxillary and mandibular swellings. The maxillary swellings are located on either side of the stomodeum, and the mandibular swellings lie caudal to it. The 2nd, 3rd and 4th arches appear as ridges on the young embryo caudal to these 1st arch structures. Each arch is composed of a core of mesoderm covered on the outside by ectoderm, and lined internally by endoderm. The arch develops its own skeletal component, which gives rise to adult bone, cartilage and ligament. Each arch has its own muscular component together with a cranial nerve to supply the muscle, and its own arterial supply from an

arch artery. The cartilage of the 1st arch consists of a dorsal portion (the maxillary process), and a ventral portion (the mandibular process, or 'Meckel's cartilage'). Both maxillary process cartilage and Meckel's cartilage, however, disappear except for two small portions at their dorsal ends. These give rise to the malleus and probably the incus in the middle ear. The mesenchyme of the maxillary process undergoes membranous ossification and forms the premaxilla, maxilla, zygomatic bone and part of the squamous temporal bone. The mandible itself forms by membranous ossification in the mesenchyme on the external surface of Meckel's cartilage. A little of Meckel's cartilage persists for some time at the symphysis menti. The sphenomandibular ligament is also a 1st arch remnant. The musculature of the 1st branchial arch develops into the muscles of mastication, and the anterior belly of digastric. The nerve supply comes from the mandibular branch of the 5th cranial nerve, which is therefore the nerve of the 1st arch.

The 2nd arch cartilage, Reichert's cartilage, gives rise to the stapes, styloid process, the stylohyoid ligament, the lesser horn and upper body of the hyoid bone. The nerve of this arch is the 7th cranial nerve, and the muscles are the muscles of facial expression, stapedius, stylohyoid, and the posterior belly of digastric. They migrate over the face and neck during development to their adult positions. The cartilage of the 3rd branchial arch gives rise to the lower part of the body and the greater horn of the hyoid bone. The only muscle associated with this arch is stylopharyngeus, and the nerve of the arch is the glossopharyngeal nerve. It is difficult to distinguish the cartilaginous components of the 4th, 5th and 6th arches, but together they form the cartilages of the larynx. Probably the only muscle associated with the 4th arch is the cricothyroid, and its nerve supply is from the external laryngeal nerve. The recurrent laryngeal branch of the vagus belongs to the 6th arch.

Development in the pharyngeal pouches gives rise to various structures in the head and neck (Fig. 7.9). The first pouch forms the tubotympanic recess which grows outwards to contact the 1st branchial cleft. The recess becomes the middle ear and auditory tube, and the 1st cleft gives rise

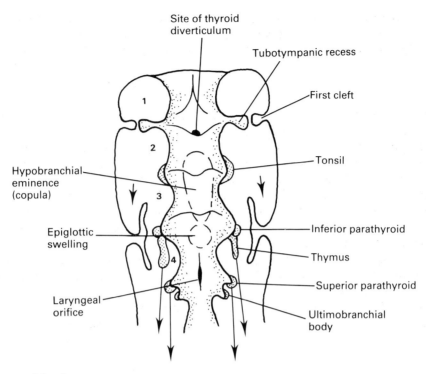

Fig. 7.9 Development of the pharynx

to the external acoustic meatus. The future tympanic membrane therefore lies between the cleft and pouch. This development is reflected in the different sensory nerve supply to the inner and outer surfaces of the membrane (see Ch. 4 and Fig. 4.1). In the depths of the 2nd pharyngeal pouch the epithelial lining proliferates and forms buds. The surrounding mesoderm invades the buds and forms the basis of the palatine tonsil. This primitive structure becomes infiltrated with lymphatic tissue during the third to fifth months of intrauterine life. The 3rd pharyngeal pouch has dorsal and ventral parts. The epithelium of the dorsal part forms a parathyroid gland and the ventral part the thymus. These structures lose connection with the pharyngeal wall and descend through the neck, the parathyroid reaching the lower posterior border of the thyroid, and the thymus reaching the mediastinum. The inferior parathyroids are therefore often referred to as 'parathyroids III'. The superior parathyroids develop in the 4th pouch and descend to their final position, and are therefore called 'parathyroids IV'. The ultimobranchial body arises from the 5th

pharyngeal pouch and becomes incorporated in the thyroid as the parafollicular or C cells. The 5th pouch degenerates; its remnants, the ultimobranchial body, and the 4th pouch are then called the 'caudal pharyngeal complex'.

Of the pharyngeal clefts, it is only the 1st cleft which forms a definitive adult structure — the external acoustic meatus. The 2nd arch tissue proliferates rapidly and overlaps the other clefts and arches. At first an ectodermal cavity remains called the 'cervical sinus', but this eventually disappears. If a sinus persists it may present as a branchial cyst or fistula. Such a cyst is located somewhere along the anterior border of sterno-cleidomastoid. On occasions there may be a fistula to the skin, and the opening is usually found low on the anterior border of sternocleidomastoid. Sometimes a complete fistula remains, the inner opening lying at the position of the 2nd pouch near the tonsil. The course of a complete fistula takes it from the skin, between the fork of the carotids to the tonsillar cleft. In this path it lies close to the 12th and 9th cranial nerves. A pre-auricular pit is probably not a form of branchial fistula.

8

THE THYROID AND PARATHYROIDS

The thyroid gland is found at the root of the neck, straddling the larynx and trachea. It lies deep to the strap muscles. The parathyroid glands, four in number, are located on the back of the thyroid gland. The surgeon is often called upon to remove part or all of the thyroid gland. This may be required as a treatment for enlargement of the gland or for malignant disease of the gland. The parathyroids also occasionally require operative exposure. Tumours of the parathyroids may occur and cause abnormalities in calcium metabolism. Such growths will need to be excised.

1. The thyroid gland

The thyroid gland consists of right and left lobes, connected across the front of the trachea by an isthmus (Fig. 8.1). The lobes are conical in shape, the apex of each rising as high as the oblique line of the thyroid cartilage. Here it is prevented from extending further upwards by the insertion of the sternothyroid muscle. Laterally, the thyroid lobe overlaps the common carotid artery and carotid sheath, and medially it lies against the inferior constrictor of the pharynx and the side of the larynx. In front of each lobe are the sternothyroid muscle, sternohyoid muscle, and the superior belly of the omohyoid. These are overlapped below by the anterior border of the sternocleidomastoid. The posterior border of the thyroid lobe is rounded, and it is here that the superior and inferior parathyroid glands may be found. The isthmus of the gland usually lies over the 2nd, 3rd and 4th tracheal rings. Occasionally, a small pyramidal lobe is found arising from the upper margin of the isthmus, or from the adjacent part of a lobe. A

fibrous band can sometimes be traced upwards from the isthmus or apex of a pyramidal lobe to the body of the hyoid bone. This is a remnant of the thyroglossal duct. Muscular tissue is occasionally found in this tract, and is called the 'levator glandulae thyroideae'.

The thyroid is completely enclosed in a fascial sheath of pretracheal fascia. The fascia at the back of the lobe is thickened to form a lateral ligament or 'ligament of Berry' which gains attachment to the cricoid cartilage (Fig. 8.2). The ligament was first described by Henle in 1883. It has also been described as having two laminae, but such a division is rarely found. There is also a looser attachment of the pretracheal fascia to the front of the trachea at the level of the isthmus. At the upper pole, the pretracheal fascia gains a firm attachment to the oblique line of the thyroid cartilage. The thyroid may also be attached to the hyoid bone by a remnant of the thyroglossal duct. These attachments of the pretracheal fascial sheath to the larynx and trachea result in movement of the thyroid gland with the larynx during the act of swallowing. A large thyroid gland or a swelling within the thyroid gland will thus move upwards during swallowing, and when a neck swelling moves in this way it is almost certain to be associated with the thyroid gland.

2. Blood supply

The thyroid is a highly vascular organ. It receives its supply from superior and inferior thyroid arteries, and sometimes from an additional source called the 'thyroidea ima'. The *superior thyroid artery* is the first branch to arise from the external

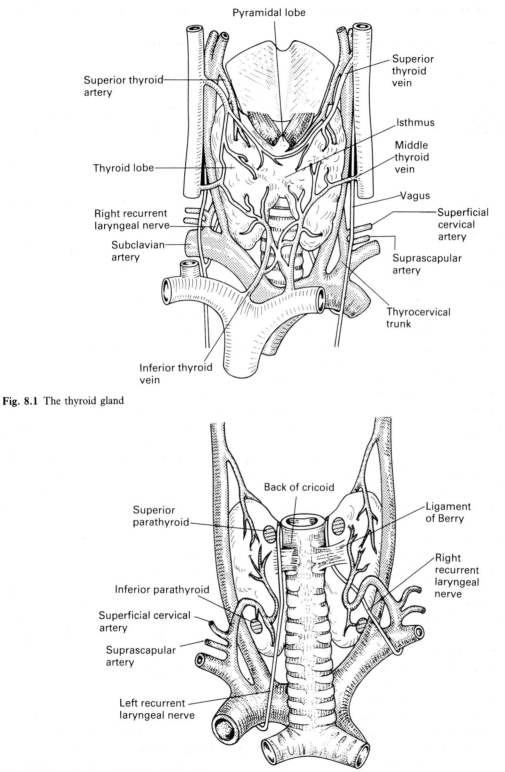

Fig. 8.1 The thyroid gland

Fig. 8.2 Posterior view of the thyroid gland

carotid artery, but on rare occasions may have an anomalous origin from the common carotid. The artery runs down the outer border of thyrohyoid and then under cover of the insertion of the sternothyroid to reach the upper pole of the thyroid lobe. Here it divides into numerous branches on the surface of the gland. In front, some branches reach the upper border of the isthmus where they anastomose with similar branches from the the opposite superior thyroid artery. Posterior branches ramify on the back of the gland and anastomose with branches of the inferior thyroid artery. The *inferior thyroid artery* arises from a stout thyrocervical trunk, a branch of the first part of the subclavian artery. The branching of the trunk is variable, but usually there are three branches — inferior

thyroid, superficial cervical, and suprascapular arteries. It is important to appreciate the course of the inferior thyroid artery in order to understand its position and relationship to the recurrent laryngeal nerve during thyroid surgery (Fig. 8.3). The artery leaves the thyrocervical trunk on the scalenus anterior, and then turns medially *behind* the carotid sheath. It therefore lies far back in the anterior compartment of the neck, just in front of the prevertebral fascia. During this part of its course it passes in front of the vertebral artery and then usually continues behind the sympathetic trunk or its middle cervical ganglion (Fig. 8.4). This latter relationship, however, is variable. The artery then descends to the lower pole of the thyroid lobe. In order to do this it has to pierce the

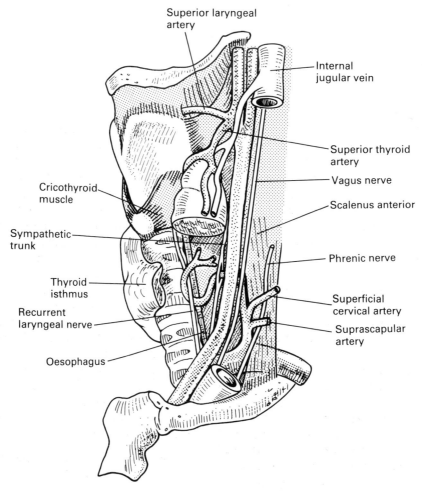

Fig. 8.3 Neurovascular relations of the thyroid gland

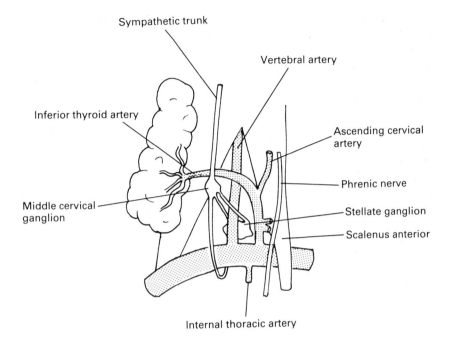

Fig. 8.4 The inferior thyroid artery

posterior pretracheal fascial sheath of the gland. The artery often gives its initial divisions before reaching the thyroid. Branches of the artery ramify on the surface of the gland and ascending branches anastomose with branches of the superior thyroid artery. Twigs from the inferior thyroid artery or its ascending branch form the principal supply to the parathyroid glands. Both thyroid arteries give arterial branches to the larynx. The superior laryngeal artery accompanies the internal laryngeal nerve, and is a branch of the superior thyroid artery (Fig. 8.3). The inferior laryngeal artery, a branch of the inferior thyroid artery, ascends to the larynx in company with the recurrent laryngeal nerve. Both superior and inferior thyroid arteries also give twigs to other adjacent structures. The superior artery gives branches to nearby muscles and the inferior artery gives pharyngeal, tracheal and oesophageal branches. An ascending cervical artery arises from the inferior thyroid artery as it lies on the scalenus anterior (Fig. 8.4). This small branch ascends close to the phrenic nerve on the surface of the muscle. The inferior thyroid artery gives spinal branches which enter the upper cer-

vical intervertebral foramina. Occasionally an *arteria thyroidea ima* arises from the aortic arch or the brachiocephalic artery and ascends in front of the trachea to reach the thyroid isthmus.

Venous drainage from the thyroid gland is collected into superior, middle and inferior thyroid veins. The superior and middle veins are paired, and enter their corresponding internal jugular vein. The inferior thyroid vein is often plexiform in nature and drains into the left brachiocephalic vein, or into both brachiocephalic veins. Lymph vessels from the thyroid communicate with a network in the capsule of the gland, and with the tracheal plexus. Lymph passes to the pretracheal and paratracheal nodes. Lymph also flows to the prelaryngeal nodes above the isthmus. Some lymph vessels descend to the brachiocephalic nodes in the superior mediastinum. Lymphatics also follow the superior thyroid vein to deep cervical nodes. Some lymph may pass directly to the thoracic duct.

3. The relationship of the laryngeal nerves to the thyroid arteries

The left recurrent laryngeal nerve ascends from

the thorax in the tracheo-oesophageal groove. Its relationship to the inferior thyroid artery in the neck is variable. Wade reported that the recurrent laryngeal nerve was deep to the artery in 50% of cases (J S Wade 1955 Vulnerability of the recurrent laryngeal nerves at thyroidectomy. *British Journal of Surgery* 43: 164–180). The surgeon may find other relationships, however, the nerve passing between terminal branches of the artery or in front of the artery (Fig. 8.5). On the right, the recurrent laryngeal nerve loops around the subclavian artery, and therefore approaches the tracheo-oesophageal groove obliquely (Fig. 8.2). It often passes between the branches of the inferior thyroid artery, but like the left, may pass in front of or behind the artery. As each recurrent nerve approaches its corresponding cricothyroid joint it has a variable relationship to the ligament of Berry. It has also been reported that the nerve may actually traverse thyroid tissue, but this is extremely rare in the normal gland. It may be useful to define Simon's triangle when locating the recurrent laryngeal nerve. The triangle has the recurrent laryngeal nerve in front, the common carotid artery behind, and the inferior thyroid artery above (see Fig. 8.7). The inferior horn of the thyroid cartilage may also serve as a guide to the recurrent laryngeal nerve.

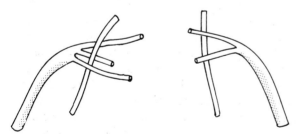

Fig. 8.5 The relations of the right and left recurrent laryngeal nerves to the inferior thyroid arteries

The external laryngeal nerve is related to the superior thyroid artery. The nerve descends on the inferior constrictor, and then passes deep to the insertion of the sternothyroid into the oblique line. The nerve often supplies the cricopharyngeal part of the inferior constrictor and may be embedded within the constrictor muscle itself. Its relationship to the superior thyroid vessels is variable, but it usually lies medial to them. The vessels, unlike the nerves, are invested in an upward prolongation of the pretracheal fascial sheath.

CASE

Bertha Bellaway, a 53-year-old housewife, had noticed a swelling in the lower neck for many years. She had been examined at the age of 40, and told that it was an enlarged thyroid gland (goitre). At that time, she was advised to have a subtotal thyroidectomy. She did not follow the advice, and presented now with a very large, multinodular goitre. There was no evidence of thyroid hyperactivity. A radiograph of the neck showed that the trachea had been compressed, and this accounted for the difficulty in breathing that she noticed. A thyroid scan showed no active nodules. Bertha was advised to undergo surgery. Following assessment and adjustment of thyroid hormone levels, Bertha was prepared for partial thyroidectomy.

Operation notes
A curved, transverse incision was made just above the hollow between the two sternal heads of the sternocleidomastoid muscles (Fig. 8.6). Such an incision heals well, and leaves very little scar. It must be remembered that there is a tendency for the scar to drop with the passage of time, and the incision was therefore not made too low. The incision was taken through the platysma to a subplatysmal plane, where dissection is relatively avascular. The upper flap of skin and platysma was dissected upwards. The deep cervical fascia was incised, and the infrahyoid strap muscles exposed. Bertha had a very large goitre, and it was therefore necessary to divide the strap muscles horizontally. The nerve supply from the ansa cervicalis usually enters the muscles at the junction of the middle and lower third. The muscles were therefore divided half-way down to avoid nerve injury. The strap muscles were dissected free of the underlying fascial capsule of the thyroid. The right lobe was rotated medially and the carotid sheath retracted laterally. This put the pretracheal fascia on the stretch, and allowed exposure of the middle thyroid vein. This was ligated and severed. This permitted medial dislocation of the gland. The upper pole of the thyroid lobe was identified, and the superior thyroid vessels carefully clamped. Care was taken not to injure the external laryngeal nerve. The vessels were doubly ligated close to the gland. With full mobilisation of the lobe, the posterior pretracheal fascia was incised, and the recurrent laryngeal nerve found in the tracheo-

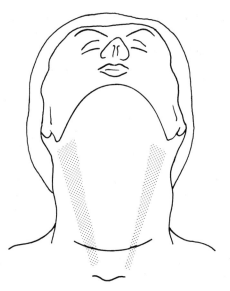

Fig. 8.6 Incision for thyroidectomy

oesophageal groove. The inferior thyroid artery was located and ligated (Fig. 8.7). Artery forceps were then clamped in a ring around the lobe and isthmus. The lobe and isthmus were excised above this protective ring. The small clamped thyroid tissue which remained was sutured to the pretracheal fascia. Leaving a little thyroid tissue in this way preserved the parathyroid glands at the back of the lobe, and left a little functioning thyroid glandular tissue. The other lobe was dealt with in a similar way. A small drain was placed deep to the strap muscles and the wound closed in layers.

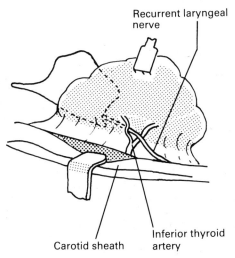

Fig. 8.7 Exposure of the inferior thyroid artery

Bertha passed the first 12 hours without incident, but suddenly developed a choking feeling and difficulty in breathing. The attendant was called, and removed the dressing from the wound. By this time Bertha had great difficulty in breathing, and the wound bulged. There had been a bleed deep to the infrahyoid strap muscles. The attendant quickly removed the skin clips and cut a deep catgut suture, and blood clot was evacuated. Bertha was returned to the operating theatre, and a small bleeding vessel was ligated. Following this emergency, she made an uneventful recovery. Postoperatively, her voice returned to normal, and both vocal cords moved normally when inspected by laryngoscopy. She had therefore not sustained injury to any of the laryngeal nerves.

4. The parathyroids

There are usually four parathyroid glands, two on each side. They are named from their positions as two superior and two inferior glands (see Fig. 8.2). Occasionally there may be more than four glands, and sometimes only three. They usually lie between the posterior borders of the thyroid lobes and the pretracheal fascial sheath, but *their exact plane is variable*. The superior parathyroid gland is more constant in position than the inferior. It is usually found on the posterior border of the lobe at the level of the lower border of the cricoid cartilage. The inferior parathyroid gland is more variable in position, and is usually more laterally placed than the superior gland, lying close to the lower pole of the thyroid lobe. Sometimes the inferior gland is found embedded in the substance of the lower pole of the thyroid. It also has a variable relationship to the inferior thyroid artery. It may, however, be found in more distant places outside the pretracheal fascial sheath of the thyroid. It may be located in front of the trachea close to the inferior thyroid veins or behind the oesophagus in the posterior mediastinum. The parathyroid glands receive a rich blood supply from the inferior thyroid arteries or from the anastomoses between these arteries and the superior thyroid arteries. Both thyroid and parathyroid glands receive a nerve supply from the sympathetic trunk, which is probably vasomotor in function.

5. Development of the thyroid and parathyroid glands

The thyroid gland may first be identified as a

thickening in the endoderm of the primitive pharynx between the 1st and 2nd arches (see Fig. 7.9
and Ch. 7). The area becomes evaginated as a midline diverticulum, which grows caudally as a tubular structure called the 'thyroglossal duct'. At
its caudal end, this bifurcates and the cells differentiate to form primary thyroid follicles. Further
subdivision results in secondary follicle formation.
The site of origin of the thyroglossal duct can be
seen on the adult tongue as the foramen caecum.
During descent of the thyroid, the thyroglossal

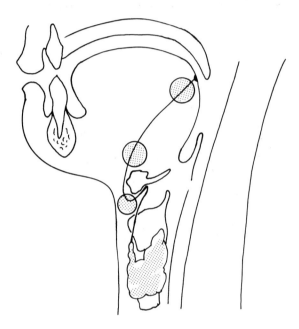

Fig. 8.8 The course of the thyroglossal duct and the
positions of aberrant thyroid tissue

duct passes first in front of the body of the hyoid
and then loops behind it before finally descending
to the front of the larynx (Fig. 8.8). Much of the
thyroglossal duct disappears, but a pyramidal lobe
represents a persistent lower part of the structure.
Occasionally aberrant masses of thyroid tissue may
be found along the course of the thyroglossal duct.
Such a mass may be found at the foramen caecum
where it forms a 'lingual' thyroid. Thyroid tissue
may also be found in relation to the hyoid. Sometimes a cystic remnant of part of the thyroglossal
duct may be found, forming a thyroglossal cyst.
Above the larynx, such a cyst is found in the midline, but cysts occurring in the lower part of the
thyroglossal duct tend to fall to one or other side of
the larynx. If a thyroglossal cyst becomes infected
and opens spontaneously or is opened surgically
onto the surface, it may form a thyroglossal fistula.
On very rare occasions thyroid tissue has been reported laterally beneath the sternocleidomastoid.
The C cells of the thyroid are derived from the ultimobranchial body.

The parathyroids are derived from the endoderm of the 3rd and 4th pharyngeal pouches. The
inferior glands (parathyroids III) develop from the
3rd pouches in close association with the thymus,
and move caudally with migration of this organ.
They stop their migration at the back of the thyroid. It can be appreciated, however, that the inferior parathyroids may on occasion end their
journey at another location on the thymus track.
The superior glands (parathyroids IV) develop
from the dorsal recesses of the 4th pharyngeal
pouches, and are more predictable in their
migration.

PART THREE

The Face

9

THE NOSE AND PARANASAL AIR SINUSES

1. The nasal cavity

The nasal cavity extends from the external nares in front to the posterior nasal apertures or 'choanae' behind, and vertically from the palate to the base of the skull. The cavity is divided into two halves by a septum. It communicates with the maxillary, frontal, ethmoidal and sphenoidal air sinuses. In front, the nose is protected by the external nose. At its root, this is formed by the nasal bones, the frontal processes of the maxillae, and the nasal part of the frontal bone. The point where the internasal and frontonasal sutures meet is called the 'nasion'. Other support for the external nose is given by lateral, major alar, and minor alar cartilages. Just inside the aperture of the nostril the cavity is dilated as the nasal vestibule and is here lined by skin, hairs, sebaceous and sweat glands.

Each half of the cavity of the nose has a lateral wall, a medial wall, a roof and a floor. The bony framework of the *lateral wall* is built from several bones. The maxilla forms a large part of the wall, and has an opening through which the maxillary air sinus communicates with the cavity of the nose. Although the opening in the maxilla is large, other bones of the lateral wall overlap the opening and reduce its effective size (Fig. 9.1). The ethmoidal labyrinth intervenes between the nasal cavity and the orbit, and on the nasal side presents two projections, the superior and middle conchae (turbinates). The superior concha is small, and overlaps the superior meatus, in which the posterior ethmoidal air cells open. The middle concha is larger and overlaps the middle meatus. If it is removed, as in Figure 9.2, a bony elevation

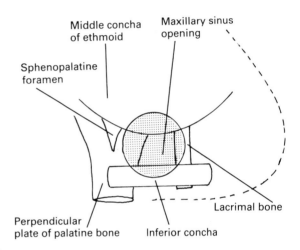

Fig. 9.1 The bones of the lateral wall of the nose

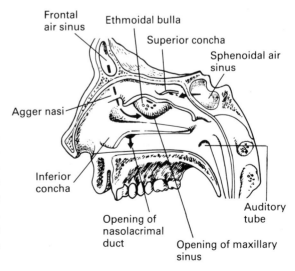

Fig. 9.2 The lateral wall of the nose

133

will be revealed, belonging to the ethmoid, called the 'ethmoidal bulla'. It is formed by the underlying middle ethmoidal air cells. The ethmoid extends from the bulla over the maxillary air sinus opening, as a flake of bone called the 'uncinate process'. The curved gutter between the uncinate process and the bulla is called the 'hiatus semilunaris', and traced forwards this leads to the infundibulum. Anterior and middle ethmoidal air cells open into the infundibulum and hiatus semilunaris. The frontal air sinus opens either into the infundibulum or directly into the middle meatus. In the living state, when the lateral wall is covered with mucous membrane, the middle meatus may be traced forwards to a depression above the vestibule called the 'atrium'. Sometimes this is limited by a curved ridge above called the 'agger nasi'.

The opening into the maxillary air sinus is overlapped below by the inferior concha, an independent bone which articulates with both maxilla and palatine bone. Overlapping the maxillary opening in front, is the delicate lacrimal bone. The nasolacrimal duct lies in an osseous canal formed by the maxilla, the lacrimal bone and the inferior nasal concha. It opens into the inferior meatus beneath the inferior concha. Behind, the maxillary opening is overlapped by the perpendicular plate of the palatine bone. This bone is Y-shaped, the two limbs of the 'Y' guarding an opening called the sphenopalatine foramen. This foramen leads from the nose into the pterygopalatine fossa behind the maxilla. The nasal bone forms part of the anterior extremity of the lateral wall of the nose.

The *medial wall* of the nasal cavity is the nasal septum. The bony part of this septum is formed below by the vomer, and the perpendicular plate of the ethmoid above. In front of these two bones the septum is cartilaginous. The septum is not always found in the midline, and may be deviated to one side or the other. Such a deviated and deformed nasal septum may block the nasal passages. The floor of the nasal cavity is formed by the upper surface of the palate. In front, are the palatine processes of the maxillae, and behind are the horizontal plates of the palatine bones. An opening in the anterior part of the floor leads into the incisive canals, which open below into the

incisive fossa on the bony palate. On each side of the septum, close to the incisive canal, is a minute orifice which represents the vestigial vomeronasal organ. This organ, well developed in lower animals in whom a keen sense of smell is essential, is rudimentary in man. The *roof* of the nasal cavity is formed by the frontal and nasal bones, and by the cribriform plate of the ethmoid. The sphenoid lies further back, with a sphenoethmoidal recess between it and the ethmoid. The sphenoidal air sinuses open into this recess.

2. The paranasal air sinuses

The *maxillary air sinuses* are pyramidal in shape. The base of each sinus forms much of the lateral wall of the nasal cavity, and the apex extends laterally to the zygomatic process of the maxilla. The roof, also part of the floor of the orbit, has the infraorbital canal running through it. The floor of the sinus is formed by the alveolar processes, and the roots of the 1st and 2nd molar teeth often raise projections in the floor of the sinus. The roots of other teeth, such as the premolars, the 3rd molars and the canines may also project into the sinus. On occasions the root of a tooth will perforate the bone and lie just beneath the mucous membrane. The maxillary air sinus opens into the hiatus semilunaris and is small in the living state. Accumulations of pus in the sinus do not drain well through the opening, for not only is it overlapped by several bones, but it also lies well above the floor of the maxillary sinus. Thus pathological fluid tends to pool in the floor of the sinus. In addition to this, pus from either infected frontal or ethmoidal sinuses may drain along the hiatus semilunaris and infect the maxillary air sinus. The maxillary air sinus is rudimentary at birth, but may be seen on a radiograph as a small slit to the medial side of the infraorbital foramen. The sinuses enlarge rapidly during the time of eruption of the permanent teeth and after puberty. This enlargement is responsible for much of the change in size and shape of the face during these periods of growth.

The two *frontal air sinuses* lie between the inner and outer tables of the frontal bone. They are rarely symmetrical, and are often separated by a septum. Their shape and size vary considerably, and one or other sinus may be absent. Like the maxillary air sinuses, they are also rudimentary or absent at birth. The *ethmoidal air sinuses* are usually divided into anterior, middle, and posterior groups. This is a fairly arbitrary division, based on the position of their openings on the lateral wall of the nose. The ethmoidal sinuses are present at birth, but are not large. They grow rapidly between the sixth and eighth years and again at puberty. The *two sphenoidal air sinuses*, like the frontal air sinuses, vary considerably in size and shape. They usually occupy the body of the sphenoid, but on occasions may extend as far as the greater wings of the sphenoid. They open into the cavity of the nose through the sphenoethmoidal recess.

3. Radiological anatomy of the facial bones and paranasal air sinuses

The bones of the face are usually examined together, but special views are needed for the nasal bones and the mandible. Several radiographic views are also required to show each of the paranasal air sinuses. Although the straight posteroanterior skull radiograph is useful, a view often used for the study of the facial bones and sinuses is made with the nose just raised off the film (Fig. 9.3). This produces in effect an occipitomental view. Further tilting to 30° places the chin directly on the film, and produces a view called the 'Waters' projection'.

The *posteroanterior view of the face, (occipitomental)* clearly shows the margins of the orbits (Fig. 9.4A). This is also a good view for examination of the frontal air sinuses, and they can be outlined as oakleaf-like translucencies above the root of the nose and orbits. They are separated by a septum above the root of the nose. This is not always in the midline, however, and the sinuses often differ in size and shape. The view is not useful for looking at the ethmoidal or sphenoidal air sinuses, for these are obscured by the nasal bones. The nasal cavity and nasal septum can, however, be seen. The view can be used for the maxillary air sinuses, for the shadows of the petrous temporal bones lie below them. Laterally, is the diamond-shaped zygomatic bone, and on the lateral orbital margin you will find the suture between this bone and the frontal bone, the fron-

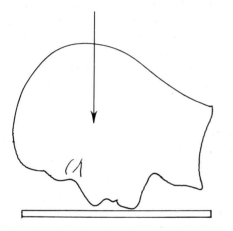

Fig. 9.3 Position of the head for radiology of the sinuses

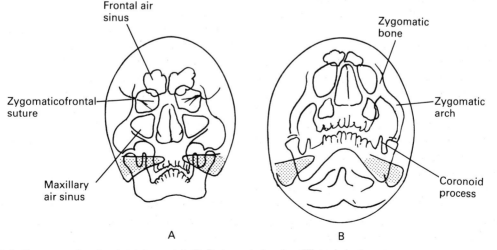

A

B

Fig. 9.4 A: Posteroanterior view (occipitomental). B: Posteroanterior view (Waters' view).

tozygomatic suture. The line made by this suture must not be mistaken for a fracture of the lateral wall of the orbit. The *posteroanterior view (occipitomental) with 30° tilt, or 'Waters' view'*, shows similar features to the previous projection (Figs. 9.4B, 9.5). Although used to show the sinuses, it is also useful for demonstrating the zygomatic bone and the zygomatic arch. The coronoid processes are also outlined in this view.

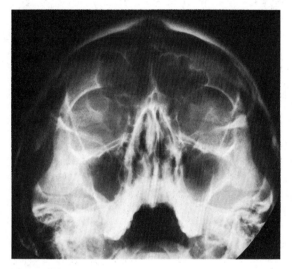

Fig. 9.5 Waters' view

This type of radiograph is therefore particularly useful in a case of suspected fracture of the zygomatic bone. The main features of the *straight occipitofrontal radiograph* of the skull are given in chapter 1 (Figs. 1.11, 1.12). This film is taken with the base line at 90° to the film, so that the shadows of the petrous temporal bones project across the orbits. Although the maxillary air sinuses are clearly visible, the lateral masses of the atlas are superimposed upon them. The view, however, gives a better picture of the floor of the maxillary air sinus and the alveolar processes than the previous two projections. The cavity of the nose is clear, together with the nasal septum. In this projection the ethmoidal and sphenoidal sinuses are superimposed, and it is therefore not useful as a view for differentiating problems in these sinuses. The projection also gives a poor view of the frontal air sinuses. The anterior ethmoidal air sinuses may be examined with a *10°*

tilted occipitofrontal radiograph. In this view the frontal air sinuses are also seen. The posterior ethmoidal and sphenoidal air sinuses can be demonstrated through the base of the skull by using a *submentovertical radiograph* (see Figs. 1.17, 1.18, 9.6). The ethmoidal sinuses will be found behind the body of the mandible on either side of the nasal septum, overlapping the sphenoidal air sinuses a little further back. A special view of the posterior ethmoidal air sinuses can be taken by making an oblique film with the line of the tube pointing at the optic foramen. This gives a clear view of the medial wall of the orbit, ethmoidal air sinuses and the optic foramen itself (see Fig. 3.2).

The *lateral radiograph of the skull* is also used to study both facial bones and sinuses (see Fig. 1.8). It gives good side views of both frontal and sphenoidal air sinuses. The extent of the frontal air sinuses is clear, especially if there is an extension into the orbital plate of the frontal bone. A lateral view of the maxillary air sinus is also given in this projection.

CASE 1

Gordon Fenwick, a 29-year-old engineer, fell while skiing in Switzerland. As he fell, he struck the left side of his face on a ski. When seen at the Alpine clinic, he was found to have a bruised and swollen left cheek. There was a subconjunctival haemorrhage in the left eye, and the lower orbital margin and maxilla were tender. Sensation over the left cheek was normal. The initial radiograph taken at the clinic did not show a fracture of the maxilla, but there was a fluid level of blood in the left maxillary air sinus (Fig. 9.7). He was therefore presumed to have a fracture involving the maxilla. It is important to examine the sinuses on radiographs of injured patients, because sometimes an opaque sinus will be the only clue to bony injury. Gordon's facial swelling subsided during the subsequent weeks, and further radiographs failed to show the fracture. The floor of the orbit was stable, and he did not develop double vision. Sensation remained normal over the cheek, indicating that the infraorbital nerve had not been damaged. The student should test for double vision and cheek sensation whenever he is presented with an injury to the front of the face. A repeat radiograph 6 weeks after the injury showed that the blood had cleared from the maxillary sinus.

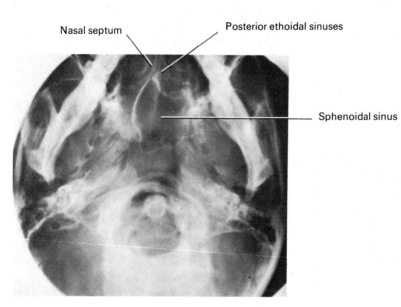

Fig. 9.6 Submentovertical view to show details of sphenoidal and posterior ethmoidal sinuses

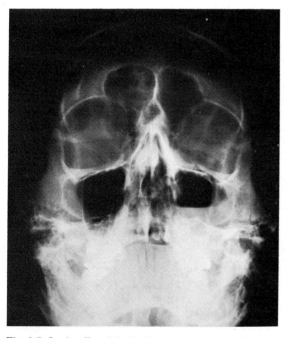

Fig. 9.7 Gordon Fenwick. Radiograph of the maxillary sinuses. (By kind permission of Mr. L. Flood FRCS and Dr P. Hamlyn, Royal Ear Hospital, London.)

CASE 2

Millie Mercury, a 40-year-old child's nurse, caught influenza from her ward. She remained in bed for a week, and then decided to start work again. She developed a severe left-sided frontal headache, and pain below the left eye. When seen at the local health centre, she had a pyrexia, and was tender over both left maxillary and left frontal sinuses. A radiograph showed that the left maxillary air sinus was completely opaque, and that there was a fluid level in the left frontal air sinus (Fig. 9.8). She was given a course of antibiotics, and made some improvement. Over the course of the next few weeks, the frontal sinusitis cleared, but the maxillary sinus remained full. Millie was referred for proof puncture and antral lavage. (The maxillary air sinus is often called the 'antrum' by the ENT surgeon.) Proof puncture was performed under a general anaesthetic. A trocar and cannula were driven through the thin bone beneath the inferior turbinate into the maxillary sinus. The trocar was removed, and a syringe attached to the cannula. Pus was aspirated and a specimen sent for culture and antibiotic sensitivity. A Higginson syringe was then attached to the cannula and the sinus washed out with sterile saline at body temperature. This procedure blew open the opening of the maxillary sinus, and washed out the sinus. At the end of the operation, a polythene tube was inserted through the cannula into the sinus and left in place. The nursing staff washed out the maxillary antrum 3 times daily for the following 2 days, by which time it was clear.

CASE 3

Samuel Pellin, a 46-year-old chronic alcoholic vagrant, presented himself at the emergency unit with a swollen and inflamed forehead. On examination, there was bony tenderness of the forehead and both maxillae. He was pyrexial. A radiograph showed that both maxillae were opaque; there was also opacity of the left ethmoidal sinuses and frontal sinuses (Fig. 9.9). The frontal bone had a 'fluffy' appearance, indicating spread of infection from the sinus to bone. He therefore had frontal osteomyelitis (inflammation of bone). He was admitted for an intensive course of antibiotics and for rehabilitation. He was discharged after 3 weeks of treatment in a reasonably fair state of health, but was seen a few weeks later in the emergency unit with hepatitis.

4. The maxillary division of the trigeminal nerve

The maxillary nerve, after leaving the trigeminal ganglion, can be traced forwards in the lateral wall of the cavernous sinus to the foramen rotundum. It leaves the cranial cavity through this foramen and enters the pterygopalatine fossa. It continues forwards to the back of the maxilla where it enters the orbit through the inferior orbital fissure. The nerve is now renamed, and called the 'infraorbital nerve'. It may be traced through the infraorbital groove or canal to emerge on the face at the infraorbital foramen.

Near the foramen rotundum, within the cranial cavity, the maxillary nerve gives a small *meningeal branch*. Several *ganglionic branches* suspend the pterygopalatine (sphenopalatine) ganglion from the nerve in the pterygopalatine fossa. The pterygopalatine ganglion is one of the four parasympathetic head ganglia, parasympathetic input arriving from the greater superficial petrosal branch of the facial nerve. The course of this branch of the facial nerve through the middle cranial fossa is described in Chapter 4. At the pterygoid canal, it joins with sympathetic fibres from the internal carotid plexus. These fibres originate in the superior

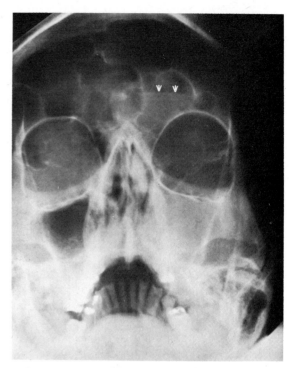

Fig. 9.8 Millie Mercury. Radiograph of the sinuses. The white arrows point to the fluid level in the frontal sinus. (By kind permission of Mr L. Flood FRCS and Dr. P. Hamlyn, Royal Ear Hospital, London.)

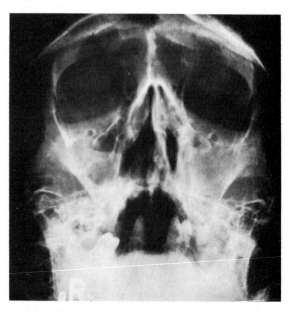

Fig. 9.9 Samuel Pellin. Radiograph of the sinuses. (By kind permission of Mr L. Flood FRCS and Dr P. Hamlyn, Royal Ear Hospital, London.)

cervical sympathetic ganglion. The mixed para-sympathetic and sympathetic bundle, called the 'nerve of the pterygoid canal', continues forwards through the canal to the pterygopalatine fossa. Only the parasympathetic fibres synapse in the ganglion; the sympathetic fibres pass through without synapse. The parasympathetic fibres are secretomotor to the lacrimal gland, and to glands in the nose, nasopharynx, paranasal air sinuses and palate. The sympathetic fibres are vasomotor in nature. Sensory fibres from the nose, sinuses and palate pass through the ganglion to the maxillary nerve, and have their cell bodies in the trigeminal ganglion. Of the branches of distribution for these mixed autonomic and sensory fibres, four sets appear to arise directly from the ganglion and one directly from the maxillary nerve itself. The branches which arise from the ganglion are described as *orbital, palatine, nasal, and pharyngeal*. The branch of distribution from the maxillary nerve itself is the *zygomatic nerve*. Orbital branches from the pterygopalatine ganglion carry parasympathetic and sympathetic fibres to a retro-orbital plexus, which supplies the orbitalis muscle and also gives a few fibres to the lacrimal gland. It also carries sensation from the orbital periosteum. The palatine branches are divided into anterior, middle and posterior groups. The anterior palatine nerve (greater palatine) descends from the ganglion through the greater palatine canal, and emerges at the greater palatine foramen of the bony palate. It supplies the gums and mucous membrane of the hard palate. During its course in the canal, the nerve gives nasal branches to the posteroinferior aspect of the lateral wall of the nose. The middle and posterior palatine nerves (lesser palatine nerves) descend through the greater palatine canal, but emerge through the lesser palatine foramina. They form a plexus with the glossopharyngeal nerve to supply sensation over the tonsil, and they also supply sensation on the soft palate. They carry taste fibres from the palate to the 7th cranial nerve, and also carry parasympathetic fibres to glands of the palate. Lateral and medial posterior superior nasal nerves stream into the lateral wall of the nose from the pterygopalatine ganglion through the sphenopalatine foramen. One of the medial posterior superior group is particularly long, and called the 'nasopalatine' (long sphenopalatine)

nerve. This runs to the nasal septum, and descends in a groove on the vomer to reach the incisive foramen in the hard palate. It is said that, when two foramina are present, the left nerve passes through the anterior foramen and the right through the posterior foramen. A pharyngeal branch of the pterygopalatine ganglion passes through the palatinovaginal canal to supply sensation to the nasal part of the pharynx, and parasympathetic fibres to mucous glands in the same area.

The zygomatic nerve arises directly from the maxillary nerve, and enters the orbit through the inferior orbital fissure. On the lateral wall of the orbit it divides into zygomaticotemporal and zygomaticofacial branches. The zygomaticotemporal branch passes through a canal in the zygomatic bone to reach the temporal fossa, and is distributed to skin on the temple. The zygomaticofacial branch also passes through a foramen in the zygomatic bone and supplies skin on the prominence of the cheek. Parasympathetic fibres reach the zygomatic nerve from the pterygopalatine ganglion, and usually enter the zygomaticotemporal branch. On the lateral wall of the orbit, they leave the nerve, and ascend as a communicating branch to the lacrimal nerve. In this way they take secretomotor fibres to the lacrimal gland.

Superior alveolar nerves arise from the maxillary and infraorbital nerves. The *posterior superior alveolar nerve* arises from the maxillary nerve itself in the pterygopalatine fossa. It pierces the infratemporal surface of the maxilla, and after supplying branches to the maxillary air sinus mucosa, forms the molar part of the superior dental plexus. This supplies sensation to the molar teeth, the adjacent part of the upper gum, and cheek. The *middle and anterior superior alveolar nerves* arise from the infraorbital nerve. The middle nerve is not always found, but when present takes part in the formation of the superior dental plexus and gives twigs to the upper premolar teeth. The anterior superior alveolar nerve runs in a sinuous canal in the anterior wall of the maxillary air sinus towards the nose. It takes part in the formation of the superior dental plexus and supplies the incisor and canine teeth. It also supplies nasal branches to the lower part of the lateral wall of the nose.

The terminal twigs of the maxillary nerve emerge at the infraorbital foramen, and are described as *palpebral, nasal, and superior labial branches*. The palpebral branches supply skin on the lower eyelid, the nasal branches skin on the side of the nose, and the labial branches skin on the front of the cheek and skin and mucous membrane of the upper lip. Injuries which result in fractures of the floor of the orbit or the maxilla sometimes also damage the infraorbital nerve (see comments in CASE 1).

5. Neurovascular supply to the nose

A summary of the sensory nerve supply to the lateral wall of the nose is given in Figure 9.10. The septum is supplied by branches of the nasopalatine and anterior ethmoidal nerves. Olfactory mucosa is limited to the upper nasal concha and adjacent parts of the septum and roof. The olfactory nerves ascend through the holes in the cribriform plate of the ethmoid. Communications exist along the olfactory nerves between the CSF and nasal lymphatics. The sensory nerve supply to the paranasal sinuses comes from the maxillary and ophthalmic divisions of the trigeminal nerve. The sensory supply to the maxillary air sinuses comes from the infraorbital nerve and from the superior alveolar nerves (Fig. 9.11). Some twigs from the anterior palatine nerve also assist in the supply. Sensation in the frontal air sinus is provided by the supraorbital nerve. The anterior and posterior ethmoidal nerves supply the ethmoidal air sinuses, and the posterior nerve also supplies sensation in the sphenoidal air sinus (Fig. 9.12). Orbital branches of the pterygopalatine ganglion assist in the sensory supply to both ethmoidal and sphenoidal air sinuses.

The arterial supply to the nose comes from branches of the ophthalmic, maxillary and facial arteries. The ethmoidal arteries assist in the supply of the mucous membrane in the roof of the nose. The sphenopalatine branch of the maxillary artery enters the nose through the sphenopalatine foramen and supplies blood to the lateral wall and the septum. The terminal part of the greater palatine artery, another branch of the maxillary artery, *ascends* through the incisive canal and anastomoses with twigs from the superior labial

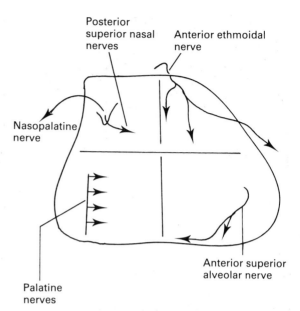

Fig. 9.10 Nerve supply to the lateral wall of the nose

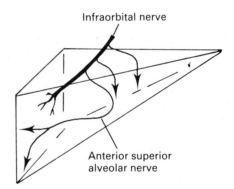

Fig. 9.11 Nerve supply to the maxillary air sinuses

branch of the facial artery in the mucous membrane of the vestibule. The most usual site for bleeding from the nose (epistaxis) is from the region of this anastomosis. The veins of the nasal cavity form a cavernous plexus beneath the mucous membrane, and veins follow the arterial pathways to regional veins.

Infection in a paranasal air sinus leads to localised pain and bony tenderness over the sinus. Infection may progress to involve the regional lymph nodes. The maxillary and frontal air sinuses

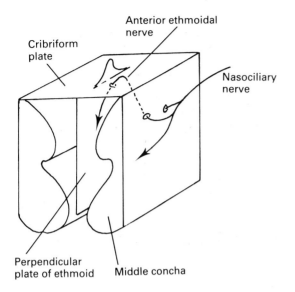

Fig. 9.12 Nerve supply to the ethmoid sinuses

further back from the right side, above the level of the middle concha. It was not controlled by the standard nasal pack. A lubricated Foley catheter was inserted into the nostril as far back as the nasopharynx. The balloon at the end of the catheter was then inflated, and the catheter pulled forwards to occlude the posterior aperture of the nose. It was strapped in place on the face. The nose was then packed as far back as the catheter. Unfortunately, when the catheter was removed, the bleeding restarted. It was decided to tie the feeding vessel to the area, the anterior ethmoidal artery. Under a general anaesthetic, the vessel was approached in the medial wall of the orbit. It was found one finger-breadth below the orbital roof, and tied. If the bleeding had been coming from below the middle concha, the maxillary artery could have been clipped in the pterygopalatine fossa. This region can be approached through the maxillary sinus. Myfanwi made a good recovery, and had no further nose bleeds. About 98% of epistaxes can be controlled by simple packing and cautery, and very few patients need to have a feeding vessel ligated.

CASE 5

Abner Blake, a 66-year-old retired nightwatchman, complained of blockage of the right side of the nose for 12 months. During recent months he had noticed a purulent discharge from the right nostril and an overflow of tears from the right eye. In recent weeks he had excruciating pain localised to the right cheek. The initial radiograph of the sinuses is shown in Figure 9.13. The right side of the nose is blocked, and the maxillary sinus is opaque. A CT scan confirmed that a large mass was present. It turned out to be a malignant tumour involving the lateral wall of the nose, with extension to the medial orbital wall, and blockage of the nasolacrimal duct. The pain was due to involvement of the infraorbital nerve. Abner underwent initial radiotherapy, followed by a radical removal of the maxilla. The deformity was covered by a prosthesis attached to a pair of spectacles. Postoperatively he made a remarkable recovery, and was pain-free.

drain to the submandibular lymph nodes, and thence to the upper deep cervical nodes. The ethmoidal and sphenoidal air sinuses have their main drainage into retropharyngeal nodes, but some lymph from the anterior ethmoidal air sinuses drains to the submandibular nodes. Lymph from the anterior part of the nasal cavity drains into the submandibular nodes, and from the posterior part of the floor into the parotid nodes.

CASE 4

Myfanwi Morgan, the 37-year-old conductor of a Welsh choir, suffered from recurrent nose bleeds. She had been seen on several occasions, and had been treated with nasal packs. She did not have a bleeding disorder, leukaemia or any other general disease likely to cause the condition. On the last occasion the bleeding site was found to be located in Little's area. This is the area of anastomosis between the sphenopalatine artery and other vessels in the anteroinferior angle of the nasal septum. This area was therefore cauterised. During a strenuous conducting effort while the choir was singing at a festival, she had a further epistaxis, and had to be taken to the nearest emergency unit. On this occasion, the bleeding was not coming from the front of the nose, but

CASE 6

Jeremy Bryton, a 37-year-old textile worker, had been troubled with sinusitis for several years. During the most recent attack, he was seen at the local health centre, where a radiograph showed an opaque right maxillary air sinus and a fluid level in the left sinus. He was treated with antibiotics with only slight clearing of the right sinus. When seen at the ENT clinic, a further radiograph was taken with the head tilted (Fig. 9.14). This showed that the line of opacity in the left sinus was not a fluid level, because its relationship to the head remained unchanged. It was a papilloma of the lining of the maxillary air sinus. At operation, the left maxillary sinus was exposed through the mouth, and the tumour excised.

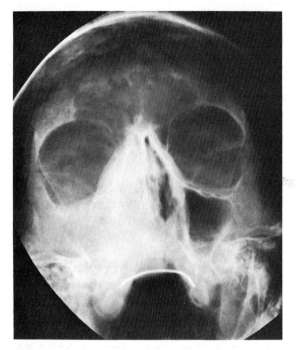

Fig. 9.13 Abner Blake. Radiograph of the sinuses. (By kind permission of Mr L. Flood FRCS and Dr P. Hamlyn, Royal Ear Hospital, London.)

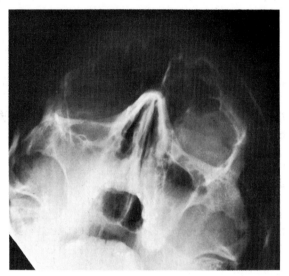

Fig. 9.14 Jeremy Bryton. Radiograph of the maxillary sinuses with the head tilted. (By kind permission of Mr L. Flood FRCS and Dr P. Hamlyn, Royal Ear Hospital, London.)

10

THE SIDE OF THE MOUTH AND PARAPHARYNX

In the section dealing with the basic topography of the neck in Chapter 5, it was noted that the side of the mouth overlapped the upper pharynx. The temporomandibular joint, ramus of the mandible, muscles of mastication, and parotid gland were therefore removed for the study of the upper neck. These structures, forming the mechanical part of the mouth and its major secretory element, must now be replaced and studied in detail. They not only form the side of the mouth but also lie to the side of the pharynx with the parapharyngeal space between them.

THE MANDIBLE AND TEMPOROMANDIBULAR JOINT

1. The mandible

The mandible and its articulation with the temporal bone at the temporomandibular joint (TMJ) supply the bony architecture for the side of the mouth. The mandible is divided for descriptive purposes into two parts. The body is the horizontal, horseshoe-shaped part of the bone, and the rami are the flat extensions at the posterior ends of the body. Two processes arise from the upper end of each ramus, and create a deep mandibular notch between them. In front, is the flat, triangular coronoid process, and behind is the condylar process. The upper end of this latter process is expanded as the head of the mandible, and the constricted portion below the head is called the 'neck of the mandible'. A small depression called the 'pterygoid fovea' is found on the front of the neck.

Several features can usually be identified on the outer surface of the body of the mandible. The line of fusion of the two halves of the mandible in early life is represented by a vertical ridge in the midline. At the lower end of this ridge is a mental protuberance with a small raised tubercle on either side of it. A little further back, below the 2nd premolar, is the mental foramen. A line made by the attachment of the buccinator can often be seen on the dry bone below the molar teeth. The outer surface of the ramus bears several ridges made by the tendinous insertions of the masseter (Fig. 10.1). The parotid salivary gland is located behind the ramus of the mandible between it and

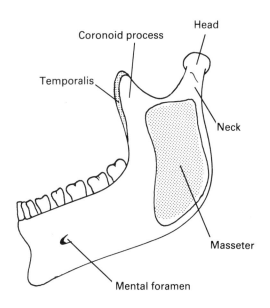

Fig. 10.1 Outer surface of the mandible

the mastoid process. From here it extends laterally over the TMJ and outer surface of the ramus, and also on to the medial aspect of the ramus. The base of the body of the mandible meets the posterior border of the ramus at the angle of the mandible (see Fig. 1.5). Here the bone is everted in the male, but inverted in the female.

The most obvious feature of the inner side of the mandible is the large mandibular foramen found in the ramus (Fig. 10.2). This leads into the mandibular canal, which passes through the body of the bone to open at the mental foramen. The mandibular foramen is guarded in front by a triangular lip of bone called the 'lingula'. A shallow groove can often be found descending from the foramen, and this is occupied by the nerve to the mylohyoid in the living state. Examination of the body will reveal an oblique ridge called the 'mylohyoid line', which marks the origin of the mylohyoid muscle. At the posterior end of the line, behind the 3rd molar tooth, is a ridge produced by the origin of the superior constrictor of the pharynx and the attachment of the pterygomandibular raphe. The mylohyoid line divides the body of the mandible into a sublingual fossa above and a submandibular fossa below. As their names suggest, the two sali-

vary glands of the floor of the mouth lie in these hollows. At the anterior end of the mylohyoid line, in the midline of the mandible, are mental spines, the upper being formed by the origin of the genioglossus and the lower by the geniohyoid. Below the anterior end of the mylohyoid line is a small fossa made by the origin of the anterior belly of the digastric. Sixteen sockets are found in the adult mandible on the upper border of the body in its alveolar part.

2. Development of the mandible

The branchial arch cartilage of the mandibular process is called 'Meckel's cartilage', but for the most part it disappears. The mandible itself forms by membranous ossification, a single centre of ossification appearing on each side during the sixth week of fetal life. It is placed well forwards, close to the mental foramen. Ossification extends in the fibrous tissue lateral to Meckel's cartilage and the inferior alveolar nerve, continues around the inferior alveolar nerve, and then upwards. The developing mandible therefore takes the form of a trough. This becomes partially partitioned to form the crypts for the developing teeth. Secondary cartilages appear, the most important of which is the condylar cartilage. This is found in the ramus of the mandible, extending to the region of the future head. It becomes ossified during fetal life, except for its uppermost portion, which remains as a disc of proliferating cartilage beneath the fibrous articular surface until the third decade of life. Other secondary cartilages are found along the anterior border of the coronoid process and on each side of the symphysis menti. In the midline, the two halves of the mandible are still united by fibrous tissue at birth, the union being called the 'symphysis menti'. During the first year of life the symphysis starts to unite from below upwards, and union is complete by the second year.

The dorsal end of Meckel's cartilage becomes separated from the developing mandible to form the malleus and possibly the incus. It has been suggested that the incus represents the quadrate bone, a structure which is a prominent feature of reptiles and earlier vertebrates. It is not much in evidence, however, in mammals. The anterior ligament of the malleus and the sphenomandibular

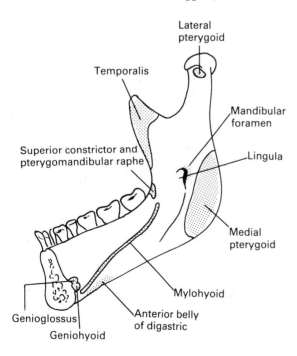

Fig. 10.2 Inner surface of the mandible

ligament are also remnants of Meckel's cartilage. The ventral end of Meckel's cartilage becomes incorporated into the developing mandible. In the newborn mandible the mandibular canal runs close to the lower border of the body of the mandible, below the sockets of the deciduous teeth. The mental foramen opens below the 1st deciduous molar tooth, and the mental nerve passes forwards through the foramen. The body elongates in particular behind the mental foramen, this growth being necessary to accommodate three additional teeth. As this occurs, and as the prominence of the chin develops, the direction of the mental foramen changes. The nerve then passes out of the foramen in a *backward* direction. The condylar cartilage, left beneath the fibrous articular covering of the head, is responsible for growth in height of the ramus, and downward and forward growth of the mandible as a whole. Remodelling continues throughout childhood, bone being laid down along the posterior borders of the coronoid process and ramus, while bone is absorbed along the anterior borders. The angle of the mandible in the newborn is obtuse, but the growth and remodelling which occurs, and the development of the teeth, result in a more acute angle in the adult. In old age, if the teeth are lost, the alveolar part of the mandible is absorbed. The mental foramen and mandibular canal lie close to the alveolar border of the body, the ramus lies more obliquely, and the angle becomes more obtuse.

3. The temporomandibular joint (TMJ)

The articulation between the head of the mandible and the temporal bone is synovial and condylar in type. The articular surfaces are unusual for synovial joints, in that they are covered with fibrous tissue containing very few cartilage cells. The articular surface of the skull consists both of the mandibular fossa and the articular eminence of the temporal bone. The fibrous capsule is attached to the circumference of the mandibular fossa and extends as far as the squamotympanic fissure behind. Below, it is attached around the neck of the mandible. The lateral side of the capsule is strengthened by fibres which extend from the tubercle on the root of the zygoma to the posterior border of the neck of the mandible. This oblique band is

called the 'temporomandibular' or 'lateral ligament'. The joint also gains support on the medial side by the sphenomandibular ligament, which stretches from the spine of the sphenoid to the lingula in front of the mandibular foramen. The stylomandibular ligament, found between the tip of the styloid and the mandibular angle, is also described as adding to the support of the joint. The capsule is lined internally by synovial membrane.

An intra-articular disc of fibrous tissue completely divides the TMJ cavity into two (Fig. 10.3). The upper surface of the disc is saddle-shaped to match the shape of the mandibular fossa and articular tubercle. The lower surface fits over the head of the mandible. The disc is attached to the capsule around its circumference. In front, fibres of the lateral pterygoid muscle insert into the capsule and into the disc, and this section of the disc is called the 'anterior extension'. The disc presents two thickened zones, the anterior and posterior bands, with a thin intermediate region between. Posteriorly, the disc becomes bilaminar, the upper lamella attaching to the back of the mandibular fossa, and the lower to the condyle. The upper lamella is composed of fibroelastic tissue, but the lower lamella is non-elastic.

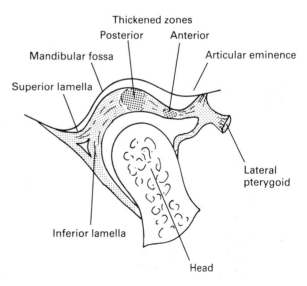

Fig. 10.3 The temporomandibular joint

4. Radiological examination of the mandible

A complete radiological examination of the mandible requires several projections, because of the recurring problem of superimposition of other structures on the mandibular shadow. In the straight posteroanterior view it is the cervical spine which is superimposed over the body of the mandible, although techniques are available to avoid loss of detail. Some features of the body of the mandible can be examined, however: the mandibular canal is visible in the body, and the lower teeth and sockets are also shown (see Fig. 1.12). The posteroanterior view is not useful for a close examination of the ramus, because this is seen in profile. The head and much of the condylar process is superimposed on the zygomatic bone shadow, and the TMJ is mostly obscured in this view. More detailed information about the posterior part of the body of the mandible and the ramus is obtained by an oblique projection (Fig. 10.4). The patient's lower jaw is placed in contact with the film, and the X-ray tube is directed obliquely upwards towards it. The ramus not under examination is projected onto the upper part of the film, giving a clear view of the ramus and body of the side in question. The upper part of the coronoid process is usually obscured by the zygomatic arch, and the angle of the mandible is overlapped by the shadow of the hyoid bone. The molar and 2nd premolar teeth and their roots are seen on this view, together with the mental foramen below the 2nd premolar tooth. The mandibular canal may be traced within the ramus and body of the mandible. If information of the mandible close to the symphysis is required, the head may be rotated so that this area is nearer the film. Special views are required to show details of the TMJ. The joint is examined by means of a lateral radiograph but the tube must be angled so that the TMJ is as free as possible of overlapping shadows (Fig. 10.5). One film should be taken with the mouth closed and the other with the mouth open. When the mouth is closed the head lies in the mandibular fossa, the joint space being fairly wide and regular because of the interposed articular disc. On the view with the mouth open, the head is found on the articular tubercle (Fig. 10.6).

CASE 1

Gertrude Summers, a nervous, 17-year-old ballet student, complained of a dull pain in the right temporomandibular joint. She stated that the pain was worse after eating, and she often noticed episodes of 'clicking' in the joint. She noticed that the joint problem was often accompanied by headache and discomfort in the ear. She was referred to a dentist

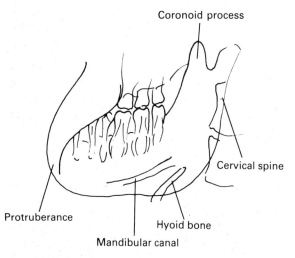

Coronoid process

Cervical spine

Protruberance

Hyoid bone

Mandibular canal

A

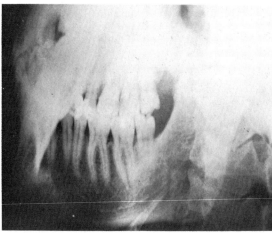

B

10.4 A: Outline of radiograph of mandible. B: Radiograph of mandible.

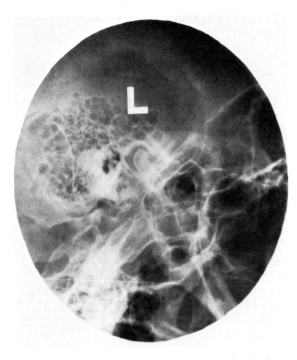

Fig. 10.5 The temporomandibular joint — mouth closed

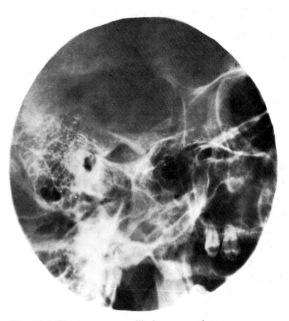

Fig. 10.6 The temporomandibular — mouth open

for examination, but was found to have normal occlusion and no problem with wisdom teeth. He could find no dental reason for the pain, but sent Gertrude for a tomogram of the TMJ. Figures 10.7 and 10.8 show the tomograms with the mouth closed and the mouth open. Such radiographs are much clearer than the straight radiographs such as those in Figures 10.5 and 10.6. The radiographs were normal. No problems were located in the ear, and the parotid gland was also normal.

It seemed that Gertrude was suffering from a pain dysfunction syndrome. This is possibly a neuromuscular coordination disturbance causing spasm and fatigue of the muscles of mastication, but the exact pathology is still not fully understood. There is also the possibility of a psychological factor in its production. It is not an uncommon condition, and best treated conservatively. Gertrude was given simple analgesics and a course of anxiolytics. She improved during the following months by these simple and supportive measures, although she still complains of 'clicking' in the joints from time to time.

5. The muscles of mastication and movements at the temporomandibular joint

The mandible may be depressed, elevated, protruded, retracted and rotated at the TMJ. This

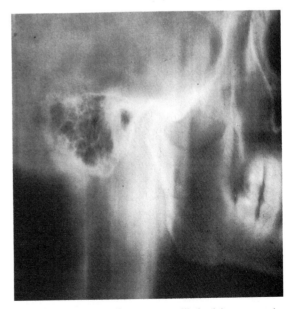

Fig. 10.7 Tomogram of temporomandibular joint — mouth closed

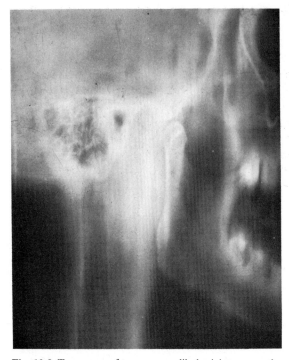

Fig. 10.8 Tomogram of temporomandibular joint — mouth open

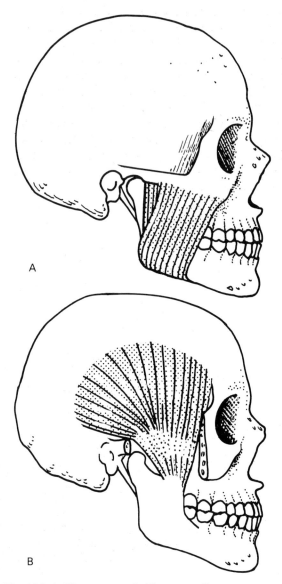

Fig. 10.9 A: The masseter. B: The temporalis.

classical description of movements, however, is an approximation. Mandibular joint movements, like those of other synovial joints, are much more complex. The mandibular head is free in reference to a sphere or envelope, movements taking it over the surface of the envelope, or within the envelope. In addition, a further set of movements may be described when the teeth are apposed, and these may be called 'contact movements'. As with other joints in the body, in spite of the more sophisticated methods of analysing joint movement, it is still useful when describing the musculature to revert to the classical nomenclature.

There are four muscles of mastication — the masseter, the temporalis, and the lateral and medial pterygoid muscles. The *masseter* extends from the zygomatic arch to the outer surface of the ramus of the mandible (Fig. 10.9A). The muscle consists of three layers, the superficial layer of which is by far the largest. It arises from the zygomatic process of the maxilla and the lower border of the zygomatic arch. Its fibres pass downwards and backwards to reach the angle and lower part

of the lateral surface of the ramus. Its insertion is partly muscular and partly tendinous, the tendinous septa raising ridges on the outer surface of the ramus. The middle and deep layers both arise from the deep surface of the zygomatic arch. The middle layer is inserted into the middle of the ramus and the deep layer into the upper part of the ramus and coronoid process. The *temporalis* is fan-shaped, and arises on its deep surface from the temporal fossa and superficially from the strong fascia which covers the muscle (Fig. 10.9B). This fascia is attached along the superior temporal line above. Below, it splits to insert into the margins of the upper border of the zygomatic arch. The fibres of temporalis converge onto a strong tendon which passes through the gap between the side of the skull and the zygomatic arch. It inserts into the apex and borders of the coronoid process and into the medial surface of the process. The anterior fibres of temporalis extend down the anterior border of the coronoid process to gain insertion close to the 3rd molar tooth.

The two pterygoid muscles are found deep to the ramus of the mandible in the parapharyngeal (infratemporal) fossa. They arise from the lateral pterygoid plate. The *lateral pterygoid* arises from the outer surface of the lateral pterygoid plate, and its fibres sweep backwards to insert into the small fovea on the front of the neck of the mandible (Fig. 10.10). It also gains insertion into the capsule of the TMJ and into its intra-articular disc. This latter insertion is of some embryological interest, for during early development the muscle inserts into the dorsal end of Meckel's cartilage, the part

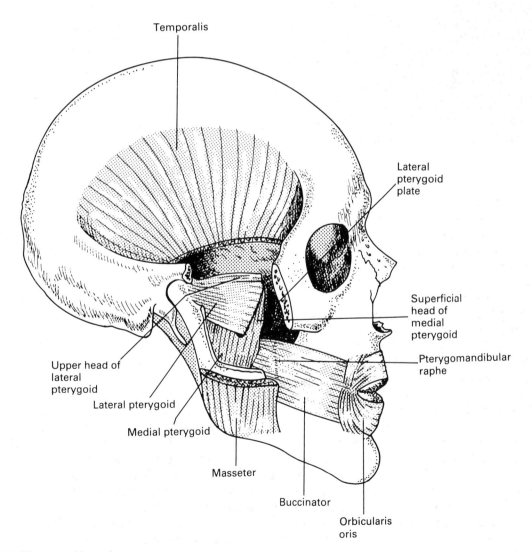

Fig. 10.10 The pterygoid muscles

which forms the malleus. Attachment to the malleus is lost, but fibres still remain attached to the disc. The lateral pterygoid has a small upper head arising from the greater wing of the sphenoid. The *medial pterygoid* arises from the inner surface of the lateral pterygoid plate, and a small pyramidal process of the palatine bone. The pyramidal process may be identified on the skull as a small projection of the palatine bone at its outer and posterior corner (see Fig. 5.3B). It wedges itself in the notch between the bases of the two pterygoid plates. The medial pterygoid fibres sweep downwards and backwards to be attached to the ramus and angle of the mandible, an attachment which is both muscular and tendinous. The medial pterygoid also has a small second head. Its origin is *superficial* to the lateral pterygoid, so that the two heads of the medial muscle clasp the lower border of the lateral pterygoid. The superficial head arises from the tuberosity of the maxilla and the pyramidal process of the palatine bone.

Both masseter and temporalis elevate the mandible. The action of the temporalis, however, is more complicated, for although the anterior fibres of this muscle exert an upward pull, the posterior fibres lie almost horizontally. They therefore have a backward pull on the mandible. This is a useful action, for when the mouth is fully open, the head of the mandible and disc sit on the articular eminence. The action of these posterior fibres therefore stabilises the bite while the mouth is wide open. They also act in pulling the head back towards the mandibular fossa. Temporalis also aids in side-to-side grinding movements. Acting alone, the medial pterygoid elevates the mandible. The lateral pterygoid, on the other hand, opens the mouth by pulling the condylar process and articular disc forwards. When the mouth is opened a small amount, this involves rotation of the head of the mandible on the articular disc. On opening the mouth widely, however, the head and disc are brought forwards to lie in contact with the articular eminence. Confirm this by feeling the head of the mandible while you open and close the mouth. The pterygoids often act together. If the medial and lateral pterygoids of one side contract, the jaw rotates about a vertical axis through the opposite condyle (Fig. 10.11). Alternate actions of this sort produce the side-to-side rotations used in grinding

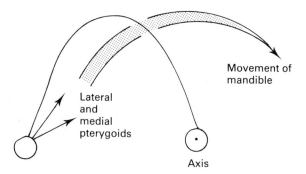

Fig. 10.11 Movement of the mandible

movements. When all four pterygoids act together, the jaw is protruded.

THE MANDIBULAR DIVISION OF THE TRIGEMINAL NERVE

The nerve of the 1st branchial arch is the mandibular division of the 5th cranial nerve (Fig. 10.12). It enters the infratemporal fossa through the foramen ovale, and has a wide distribution to the muscles of mastication, the teeth and gums, and to the skin of the face, ear and temple. It also carries ordinary and special sensation to the front of the tongue. The motor root of the mandibular nerve unites with the large sensory root below the foramen ovale. Here the mandibular nerve lies deep to the *lateral* pterygoid muscle. Medially, it lies against the tensor veli palatini, with the otic ganglion between the main trunk of the nerve and the muscle. Two branches arise from the main trunk of the mandibular nerve, a *meningeal branch*, and the *branch to the medial pterygoid*. The meningeal branch (nervus spinosus) enters the cranial cavity through the foramen spinosum in company with the middle meningeal artery. Like the artery, it divides into anterior and posterior divisions and supplies dura in the anterior and middle cranial fossae. It also supplies sensation to the mucous membrane of the mastoid air cells. The branch to the medial pterygoid gives a few filaments, which, after passing directly through the otic ganglion, supply tensor tympani and tensor veli palatini.

The mandibular nerve divides into anterior and posterior trunks. The anterior trunk supplies the

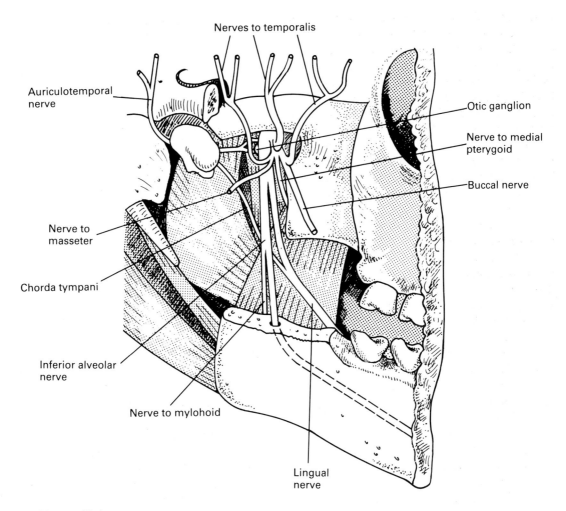

Nerves to temporalis

Auriculotemporal nerve

Otic ganglion

Nerve to medial pterygoid

Buccal nerve

Nerve to masseter

Chorda tympani

Inferior alveolar nerve

Nerve to mylohoid

Lingual nerve

Fig. 10.12 The mandibular nerve

muscles of mastication (with the exception of medial pterygoid), and gives one sensory branch, the buccal nerve. The position of these nerves should be noted. The *masseteric nerve* emerges from above the lateral pterygoid muscle and passes in front of the TMJ, behind the tendon of temporalis. It emerges through the mandibular notch with an artery, and enters the deep surface of the masseter. There are usually two *deep temporal nerves* which also emerge above the upper border of the lateral pterygoid muscle. They enter the deep surface of the temporalis. The *nerve to the lateral pterygoid* enters the deep surface of the muscle. The *buccal branch* is a long nerve which

passes between the two heads of lateral pterygoid, and emerges at the anterior border of the masseter to supply sensation to skin on the cheek and mucous membrane on the inner side of the cheek. It also supplies the adjacent buccal surface of the gum. Variations may be found in the nerve supply to the muscles of mastication, and the student must not be surprised to find other patterns of distribution.

The posterior trunk of the mandibular nerve is mostly sensory. Its motor component supplies muscles in the floor of the mouth. The trunk divides into three branches — auriculotemporal, lingual and inferior alveolar nerves. The *auriculo-*

temporal nerve is peculiar in that it usually arises by means of two roots which encircle the middle meningeal artery (Fig. 10.13). The nerve passes between the sphenomandibular ligament and the neck of the mandible to reach the posterior aspect of the TMJ. Here, it is closely related to the upper part of the parotid gland. It ascends over the zygoma to divide into anterior auricular branches, branches to the external acoustic meatus, and superficial temporal branches. The anterior auricular branches supply only skin on the tragus. The branches to the meatus supply skin in the meatus and much of the outer surface of the tympanic membrane. Temporal branches supply skin in the temporal region. The nerve also supplies articular twigs to the TMJ. The auriculotemporal nerve receives filaments from the otic ganglion. This ganglion, one of the four parasympathetic head ganglia, receives preganglionic parasympathetic fibres from the lesser petrosal nerve. This branch arises from the tympanic plexus within the middle ear, and is composed of both glossopharyngeal and facial nerve fibres, with glossopharyngeal fibres predominating. The nerve enters the parapharyngeal fossa with the mandibular nerve through the foramen ovale. The parasympathetic fibres synapse in the otic ganglion and

postganglionic fibres hitch-hike for a short distance along the auriculotemporal nerve before entering the parotid. They are secretomotor to the gland. Sympathetic fibres reach the otic ganglion from the plexus around the middle meningeal artery. They pass directly through the ganglion and also use the auriculotemporal nerve to reach the parotid. They are vasomotor in function. The otic ganglion is unique among the head ganglia in that it also transmits motor filaments. These arise from the nerve of the medial pterygoid, and innervate tensor tympani and tensor veli palatini. They do not synapse in the ganglion. Damage to the auriculotemporal nerve sometimes occurs during operations on the parotid gland or the side of the neck (see Ch. 12). This may cause sensory loss and also deprive the parotid gland of its secretomotor fibres. Fibres of the auriculotemporal nerve communicate with branches of the facial nerve. Indeed, many communicating fibres will be found between sensory nerves in the face and the facial nerve.

The *lingual nerve* is a sensory branch which carries ordinary sensation and taste to the anterior two-thirds of the tongue, in front of the sulcus. The taste fibres belong to the facial nerve. It also supplies sensation in the floor of the mouth and the mandibular gums. Soon after arising from the posterior trunk, it is joined by the chorda tympani branch of the facial nerve. The nerve carries a mixture of taste and parasympathetic fibres to the lingual nerve. The lingual nerve emerges at the lower border of the lateral pterygoid muscle, just in front of the inferior alveolar nerve. It passes forwards between the medial pterygoid and mandible to reach the lower border of the superior constrictor. A glance at Figure 10.2 will show the insertion of the superior constrictor and the pterygomandibular raphe behind the 3rd molar tooth. The lingual nerve therefore lies against the deep surface of the mandible on the medial side of the roots of the 3rd molar tooth. The further course of the lingual nerve is described in Chapter 11. The *inferior alveolar (dental) nerve* also emerges at the lower border of the lateral pterygoid muscle to pass between the sphenomandibular ligament and the ramus of the mandible. Here it reaches the mandibular foramen. Just before entering the foramen the nerve gives a mylohyoid branch, which pierces the

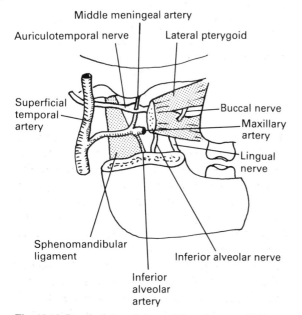

Middle meningeal artery

Auriculotemporal nerve

Lateral pterygoid

Superficial temporal artery

Buccal nerve

Maxillary artery

Lingual nerve

Sphenomandibular ligament

Inferior alveolar nerve

Inferior alveolar artery

Fig. 10.13 Detail of the relations of the sphenomandibular ligament

ligament and, grooving the medial side of the ramus of the mandible, descends to the undersurface of the mylohyoid. It supplies the anterior belly of the digastric as well as the mylohyoid. The inferior alveolar nerve itself enters the mandibular canal. The canal runs through the body of the mandible, and divides beneath the roots of the 1st and 2nd premolars into mental and incisive canals. In the adult, the mental canal curls backwards to the mental foramen, while the incisive canal continues forwards to the region of the roots of the incisor teeth. Although accounts usually describe one canal, there are often several passageways, so that the inferior alveolar nerve appears plexiform within the mandible. The incisive branch supplies the canine and incisor teeth. The mental nerve supplies skin and mucous membrane of the lower lip. Twigs from the mental nerve also form a plexus on the outer surface of the mandible to assist in supply to the incisor teeth. The teeth of the lower jaw also receive a sensory input from twigs of adjacent nerves, which enter the mandible directly. An inferior alveolar nerve block therefore does not always completely abolish sensation in the lower teeth.

CASE 2

Erik Schlomm, a 34-year-old diamond cutter with an international jewellery firm, noticed several lancinating stabs of pain in the right cheek one day while working. They were severe enough to stop him working. They recurred after a few hours, and he suffered a more prolonged paroxysm that evening. He was awoken again during the night. He consulted a physician the following day, and was told that he had trigeminal neuralgia (tic douloureux). This is a painful neuralgia of unknown origin affecting the mandibular or maxillary divisions of the 5th nerve. The ophthalmic division is rarely affected. He was referred to a neurologist. No abnormal neurological signs were found, but he was sent for a magnetic resonance imaging (MRI) scan. This showed a lesion in the pons (Fig. 10.14). Later the lesion was identified as part of the general condition of multiple sclerosis. The paroxysms of pain became frequent and long-lasting, so it was decided to inject the mandibular nerve with alcohol. Although this results in anaesthesia of the skin over the cheek and mandible, it was the only method of controlling the pain. The foramen ovale was approached by a needle inserted at the centre of the zygomatic arch and then directed towards the pterygoid plate. The needle was then withdrawn slightly, and directed backward to lie close to the mandibular nerve at the foramen ovale. If the symptoms of trigeminal neuralgia had not been localised, the trigeminal ganglion could have been approached surgically, and the sensory division sectioned. Care must be taken, however, not to affect the ophthalmic division, because corneal sensation will be lost. Eric was suffering from a widespread nervous disease, and although the mandibular pain was relieved by the injection, he had other neurological disorders from multiple sclerosis in subsequent years.

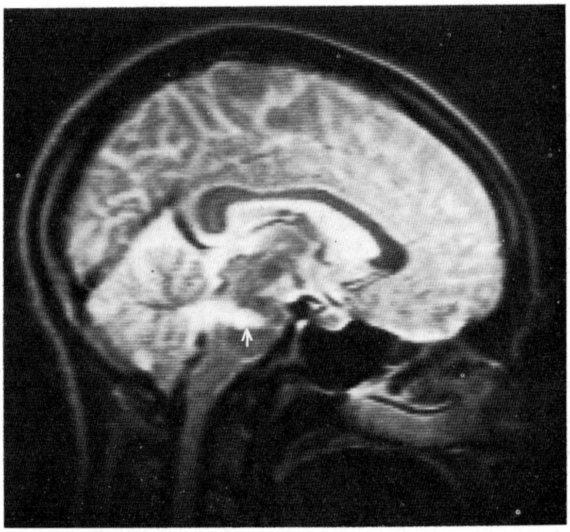

Fig. 10.14 Erik Schlomm. MRI scan showing a lesion in the pons. (By kind permission of The Multiple Sclerosis Society MRI Installation, National Hospital, Queen Square, and Professor W. I. McDonald.)

THE MAXILLARY ARTERY

The maxillary artery is one of the terminal branches of the external carotid. It arises behind the neck of the mandible, continues between the neck and sphenomandibular ligament, and then between the two heads of the lateral pterygoid. It finally enters the pterygopalatine fossa through the pterygomaxillary fissure. Although a number of branches are described, the student should only concentrate on a few of these. The *middle meningeal artery* is obviously an important branch for study. It ascends between the two roots of the auriculotemporal nerve to reach the foramen spinosum (Fig. 10.13). Its course within the cranial cavity is described in Chapter 1. An accessory meningeal branch may also arise from the maxillary artery and enter the cranial cavity through the foramen ovale. The maxillary artery gives a *branch which accompanies the inferior alveolar nerve* into the mandibular canal, and vessels which accompany the *muscular branches* of the mandibular nerve. In the pterygopalatine fossa it gives an artery which accompanies the infraorbital nerve, the posterior superior alveolar nerve and the branches of the pterygopalatine ganglion. Of these, it is important to note the posterior nasal branches to the lateral wall of the nose, for these anastomose with branches of ethmoidal arteries and the greater palatine artery. Another branch worthy of note is the *sphenopalatine artery*. This branch is, in effect, the termination of the maxillary artery. It passes through the sphenopalatine foramen into the lateral wall of the nose. It arches over the roof of the

nasal cavity, on the undersurface of the sphenoid, and reaches the nasal septum. Here it gives septal branches, one of which descends in a groove on the vomer to reach the incisive canal. The artery anastomoses with terminal branches of the greater palatine artery, and with the septal branch of the superior labial branch of the facial artery. The region of the anastomosis is called 'Little's area', and is located in the anteroinferior aspect of the septum. Epistaxis commonly results from bleeding in the region of this anastomosis.

THE PAROTID GLAND

The parotid gland clasps the back of the ramus of the mandible. It extends onto the surface of the mandible and masseter, and overlaps the posterior belly of the digastric (Fig. 10.15). The gland is

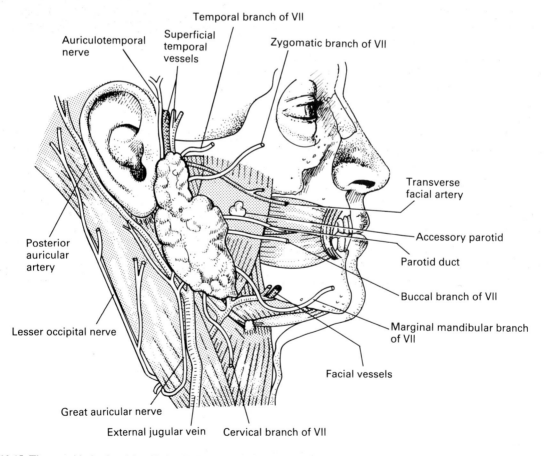

Fig. 10.15 The parotid gland and its relationships

invested in a capsule formed from deep cervical fascia. This is closely adherent to the superficial surface of the gland and attached above to the zygomatic arch. The deep part of the capsule gains attachment to structures in the parapharyngeal fossa, namely the 'styloid process' and the 'mandibular angle'. The fascia between these two points is thickened to form the stylomandibular ligament, which intervenes between the parotid and submandibular glands. At the upper extremity, the parotid forms a small extension which is closely related to the cartilaginous part of the external acoustic meatus. It lies behind the temporomandibular joint, in close relationship to the auriculotemporal nerve. The superficial surface of the gland is related to the branches of the great auricular nerve, a fact which becomes important during parotid surgery (see Ch. 12). Superficial parotid lymph nodes are also found on the surface of the gland. The parotid extends forwards onto the masseter where the parotid duct emerges. The duct passes forwards, pierces the buccinator, and opens opposite the crown of the upper 2nd molar tooth. Just above the parotid duct, on the masseter, is a small detached portion of salivary gland called the 'accessory part of the parotid gland'. The parotid extends around the back of the mandible to the styloid process and its associated muscles. This separates the gland from the internal carotid artery and internal jugular vein. The posteromedial surface of the gland is moulded against the mastoid process, sternocleidomastoid and the posterior belly of the digastric. The facial nerve, retromandibular vein and external carotid arteries pass through the substance of the parotid. Their relationship to the gland, important in parotid surgery, is outlined in detail in Chapter 12. The duct system of the gland may be examined by a radio-graph taken after injection of contrast into the parotid duct. Such a radiograph is called a 'parotid sialogram' (Fig. 10.16).

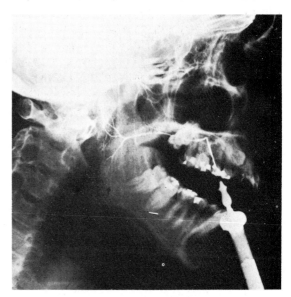

Fig. 10.16 A parotid sialogram

CASE 3

Adolph Hall, a 70-year-old caretaker of a block of apartments, noticed a swelling of the right side of his face. This became painful. When seen, the parotid was generally enlarged and tender. He was at first thought to have parotiditis, and was treated with a course of antibiotics. When the general inflammation of the gland had subsided, however, a discrete, firm lump was evident within the gland. A sialogram showed a normal duct system, and no parotid stones. The swelling proved to be a parotid tumour, and surgical removal was advised. The case history is continued in Chapter 12 together with the details of the operation of parotidectomy.

11

THE FLOOR AND ROOF OF MOUTH, THE TEETH AND SWALLOWING

THE FLOOR OF THE MOUTH AND THE TONGUE

The floor of the mouth takes the form of a muscular hammock, slung between the mandible and hyoid bone. Both of these bones are mobile. The movements of the mandible, described in Chapter 10, are elevation, depression, retraction, protrusion, and rotation. The hyoid bone can also be elevated, depressed, brought forwards and retracted but whereas the mandible is stabilised by its TMJ articulations, the hyoid bone has no such articular stability. The hyoid is like a child's swing, the ropes being the stylohyoid ligaments. It is held by muscular action which both moves and fixes the bone. Muscular fixation is necessary for the proper function of the tongue. A number of muscles are found in the floor of the mouth. The muscle which forms the hammock is the mylohyoid, but other muscles concerned with hyoid movement give additional support to the floor, and are collectively called the 'suprahyoid muscles'. Much of the extrinsic musculature of the tongue sprouts from the mandible and hyoid bone, and is supported by the floor muscles.

1. The hyoid bone

The hyoid bone is horseshoe in shape, and lies at the junction of the floor of the mouth and the neck. It is suspended from the tips of the styloid processes by stylohyoid ligaments. It is composed of a body, a pair of greater cornua and a pair of lesser cornua. The body is quadrilateral in shape, and is separated from the epiglottis behind by the thyrohyoid membrane; a bursa intervenes between the bone and the membrane. During development of the thyroid, the thyroglossal duct is closely related to this part of the bone. The greater cornua project backwards from the body, and are attached to it by cartilage, but this usually ossifies during middle life. The lesser cornua are a pair of small projections in the angles between the body and greater cornua. They are united with the body by fibrous tissue, and sometimes with the greater cornua by small synovial joints. The lesser cornua do not start to ossify until puberty. The hyoid bone is derived from the cartilage of both 2nd and 3rd branchial arches. The lesser cornua and part of the body belong to the 2nd arch and the greater cornua and lower body to the 3rd arch.

2. The muscular floor

The *digastric and stylohyoid muscles* are the two most superficial muscles to be seen when the floor of the mouth is examined from below (Fig. 11.1). The digastric muscle has two bellies united by an intermediate tendon. The posterior belly is attached to the mastoid notch of the temporal bone, and the anterior belly to the digastric fossa on the lower margin of the mandible. The two bellies are united by a rounded tendon which perforates the insertion of the stylohyoid, and is held close to the greater cornu of the hyoid bone by a fibrous loop. The stylohyoid arises from the back of the styloid process and inserts into the body of the hyoid bone. Close to the muscle is the stylohyoid ligament running from the tip of the styloid process to the lesser cornu of the hyoid. This ligament is a derivative of the cartilage of the 2nd branchial

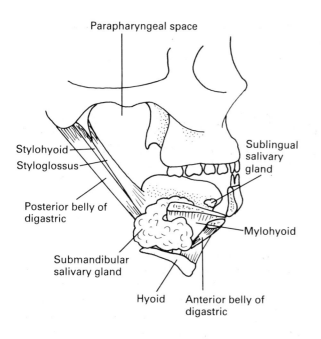

Fig. 11.1 The submandibular salivary gland

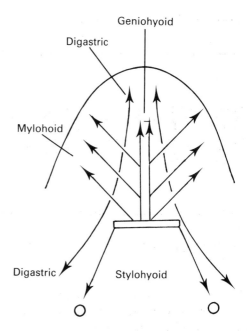

Fig. 11.2 Muscle action on the hyoid bone

arch, and is occasionally ossified. On a plane deep to the digastric and stylohyoid is the muscular hammock, the *mylohyoid* muscle. The muscle arises on each side from the mylohyoid line of the mandible, and the fibres slope posteriorly and downwards to intersect in a median raphe and insert into the hyoid bone. On the upper surface of the muscle, close to the midline is the *geniohyoid*. Lying in contact with its partner at the midline, this narrow muscle arises from the inferior mental spine, and passes backwards to the body of the hyoid bone (see Fig. 11.3).

The suprahyoid muscles move the hyoid bone, as well as forming the muscular hammock of the floor of the mouth. Their actions on the hyoid bone are summarised in Figure 11.2. The digastric and mylohyoid elevate the hyoid bone. The mylohyoid, however, does more than raise the hyoid bone, for it also supports the tongue and elevates the floor of the mouth during the first stage of deglutition. Both digastric and mylohyoid can assist in opening the mouth by depressing the mandible. Stylohyoid not only elevates the hyoid, but also draws it back. The geniohyoid elevates and draws the hyoid bone forwards. Acting in con-

junction with the infrahyoid muscles, the suprahyoid muscles can fix the hyoid bone. This is necessary for the proper function of the extrinsic tongue musculature.

3. The tongue muscles

The tongue consists of extrinsic and intrinsic musculature, the intrinsic muscles having no attachment outside the tongue. The tongue is divided into right and left halves by a midline fibrous septum which separates the muscles of the two sides. The *intrinsic musculature* is arranged longitudinally, transversely and vertically within the substance of the organ. The superior longitudinal muscle is a thin band of fibres located immediately deep to the mucous membrane of the dorsum of the tongue. It is attached behind to the epiglottis. The inferior longitudinal muscle is a band on the under-surface, extending from the root of the tongue to its apex. It lies between the genioglossus and hyoglossus. The transverse muscle of the tongue arises on each side from the median fibrous septum, and its fibres pass laterally to the sides of the organ where they blend with the fibres of the palatopharyngeus. Vertical musculature extends from dorsal to ventral surfaces of the tongue.

If the suprahyoid muscles are removed, the extrinsic muscles of the tongue are revealed (Fig. 11.3). They are the styloglossus, hyoglossus, chondroglossus, and genioglossus. The *palatoglossus* is also described as an extrinsic muscle of the tongue, but its function lies more with the palate than the tongue, for it closes off the opening between the mouth and the pharynx. In addition, its nerve supply is the same as the palatine musculature. It is therefore described later in this chapter with the palatine muscles. When the extrinsic muscles approach the tongue, they mingle with intrinsic muscle fibres. The *styloglossus* is a small muscle arising from the front of the styloid process close to its apex. Some of its fibres sweep longitudinally along the side of the tongue near its dorsal surface. Others, decussate amongst fibres of hyoglossus. The *hyoglossus* is quadrilateral in shape, and arises from the greater cornu and body of the hyoid bone. Its fibres pass vertically upwards to enter the side of the tongue deep to the styloglossus. Deep to the hyoglossus, a small bundle of muscle arises from the small lesser cornu of the hyoid bone and passes upwards into the tongue. This bundle is described as the *chondroglossus*. The *genioglossus* is a large fan-shaped muscle which arises from the upper genial tubercle on the inner surface of the mandible. Its fibres sweep downwards to the body of the hyoid and into the tongue where it enters the whole length of the ventral surface of the organ.

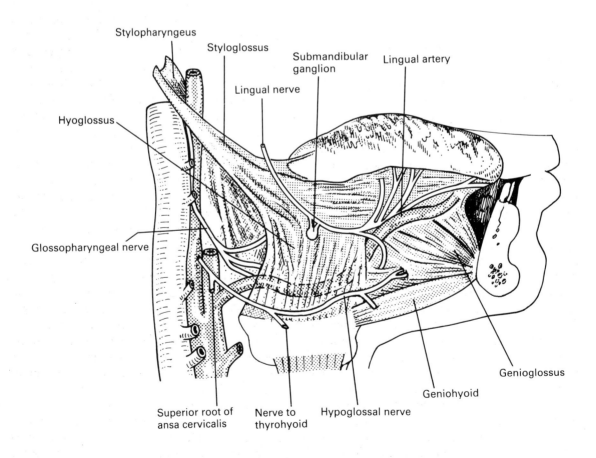

Fig. 11.3 The floor of the mouth

Movement of the tongue is complicated; it can alter its shape as well as move within and without the oral cavity. Styloglossus is able to draw the tongue backwards and upwards. Hyoglossus and chondroglossus, on the other hand, depress the tongue. The genioglossus draws the tongue forwards and protrudes it from the mouth. Genioglossus can, however, also alter the shape of the tongue. The two muscles do this by drawing the median part of the tongue downwards so that the upper surface of the tongue becomes concave from side to side. Most alteration in shape, however, is produced by the intrinsic musculature. The longitudinal muscles are used to shorten the tongue. The superior muscle aids genioglossus in producing a concave tongue, and it also draws up the tip of the tongue. Vertical musculature flattens and broadens, while the transverse muscle narrows and elongates the organ.

4. The neurovascular supply to the floor of the mouth and the tongue

Three nerves may be followed into the floor of the mouth, the nerve to the mylohyoid, the lingual nerve, and the hypoglossal nerve. The nerve to mylohyoid and the lingual nerve emerge from the parapharyngeal fossa, the former being a branch of the inferior alveolar nerve and the latter a branch of the mandibular nerve. After piercing the spheno-mandibular ligament, the *nerve to mylohyoid* descends in a groove on the medial surface of the ramus of the mandible. It passes below the mylohyoid to supply it and the anterior belly of the digastric. The posterior belly of the digastric is supplied by the 7th cranial nerve. The dual nerve supply to this muscle reflects its embryological origin from two branchial arches, the anterior belly from the 1st branchial arch and the posterior belly from the musclature of the 2nd arch. The *lingual nerve* enters the mouth on the deep surface of the mandible close to the roots of the 3rd lower molar tooth, and in this part of its course it is only covered by mucous membrane. It then passes on to the superficial surface of the hyoglossus muscle, deep to the mylohyoid (Fig. 11.3). From here, it passes forwards on to the genioglossus where it divides into its terminal branches. While on

hyoglossus it is closely related to the submandibular duct. Branches of the lingual nerve supply mucous membrane in the floor of the mouth, the lingual surface of the lower gums and general sensation to the mucous membrane of the tongue in front of the sulcus terminalis. It also supplies taste buds in this area of the tongue. The taste fibres, however, only pass along the lingual nerve for a short distance, for they leave by the chorda tympani for the facial nerve, and have their cell bodies in the genicular ganglion. The chorda tympani also transmits preganglionic parasympathetic fibres from the facial nerve. These enter the lingual nerve and hitch-hike as far as the floor of the mouth where they leave the nerve and enter the submandibular ganglion. This ganglion, one of the four parasympathetic head ganglia, appears to be suspended from the lingual nerve as it lies on the hyoglossus. After synapse, postganglionic parasympathetic secretomotor fibres pass to the submandibular gland. Other postganglionic fibres return to the lingual nerve to be carried into the floor of the mouth to supply sublingual and anterior lingual glands. Sympathetic fibres, originating from the superior cervical ganglion, form a plexus around the facial artery and send postganglionic fibres through the submandibular ganglion without synapse. These are vasomotor to the blood vessels of the salivary glands.

The *hypoglossal nerve* reaches the floor of the mouth from the neck. In the submandibular region it lies on the superficial surface of the hyoglossus below the lingual nerve. Like the lingual nerve, it also passes onto genioglossus and then continues on the muscle as far as the tip of the tongue. Hitch-hiking 1st cervical fibres leave the hypoglossal nerve as the superior root of the ansa cervicalis, and as twigs to the thyrohyoid and geniohyoid. Apart from these fibres, the hypoglossal fibres proper are distributed to the styloglossus, hyoglossus, genioglossus and the intrinsic muscles of the tongue. The hypoglossal nerve lies superficially in the side of the neck, and injury may affect both muscles of the tongue and infrahyoid musculature if its cervical fibres are damaged. If one hypoglossal nerve is injured and the subject asked to protrude the tongue, the organ deviates *to the side of the lesion*, because of the unopposed action of the opposite genioglossus. If the infrahyoid muscles are affected by loss of cervical fibres, the larynx *deviates to the unaffected side* when the subject attempts to swallow. Unilateral hypoglossal nerve injury is surprisingly not a great disability, but bilateral hypoglossal nerve injury is a most serious condition, for the act of swallowing is extremely difficult.

The *lingual artery* arises from the external carotid opposite the tip of the creater cornu of the hyoid bone. It passes close to the middle constrictor of the pharynx, and continues towards the posterior border of hyoglossus. In this part of its course the artery has a characteristic upward loop. The artery, unlike the lingual nerve, passes deep to the hyoglossus and then skirts the upper border of the hyoid cartilage. Near the anterior border of the hyoglossus, it gives dorsal lingual branches which ascend to the back of the tongue, palatoglossal arch and tonsil. It also supplies a sublingual artery to the sublingual gland and the floor of the mouth. The main part of the lingual artery ascends sharply on the side of the frenulum to the under-surface of the tongue. Here, accompanied by the lingual nerve, it is called the 'deep artery of the tongue'. Within the tongue it runs lateral to genioglossus, and at the tip of the tongue it anastomoses with the artery of the opposite side.

The tongue possesses rich lymphatic networks in both its mucous membrane and amongst its muscles. In front of the sulcus, lymph drains to marginal and central vessels. Lymph from the tip of the tongue and the frenulum drains into the marginal vessels which *may cross the midline* to reach submental nodes of the opposite side. Indeed, efferent vessels from the submental nodes may also cross the midline. The vessels reach the submental nodes by piercing the mylohyoid, very close to its origin from the mylohyoid line. One vessel usually runs beyond the submental nodes to reach the jugulo-omohyoid node. Further back, on the anterior two-thirds of the tongue, lymph vessels pass from the marginal vessels, in close relationship to the sublingual salivary gland, through the origin of mylohyoid to the submandibular nodes. A few of these may reach the jugulodigastric and jugulo-omohyoid nodes. Some vessels accompany the hypoglossal nerve as far as the jugulodigastric node. Some vessels drain directly from the posterior tongue margin, through the pharyngeal wall, into the jugulodigastric node. The central vessels are located between the genioglossi. From here they follow the lingual vessels to the deep cervical nodes, especially to the jugulodigastric and jugulo-omohyoid. They may pass along the vessels of the opposite side to lymph nodes on the other side of the neck. Lymph vessels from the posterior third of the tongue and the vallate papillae may also pass to both sides of the neck. They pierce the pharyngeal wall and reach the deep cervical nodes, in particular the jugulodigastric and jugulo-omohyoid nodes. One vessel often emerges through the thyrohyoid membrane and ends in the jugulo-omohyoid node. From the above account, it can be seen that a carcinoma of the tongue may show lymph node involvement in the submental, submandibular, or in nodes of the deep cervical chain. Of these latter nodes, the jugulo-omohyoid is particularly likely to be involved. A lesion on one side of the tongue may result in node involvement on the opposite side of the neck.

5. Salivary glands in the floor of the mouth

The submandibular and sublingual salivary glands are two large salivary glands in the floor of the mouth, but accessory glands are also found in the mouth, on the tongue, tonsil, soft and hard palates, and on the surfaces of the lips and cheeks. The *submandibular salivary gland* lies in the submandibular fossa on the inner side of the mandible. Here it clasps the lateral edge of the mylohyoid muscle, which therefore partially divides it into superficial and deep parts (see Fig. 11.1). The superficial part lies on the surface of mylohyoid, and the deep part extends above the muscle in the cleft between it and hyoglossus. The gland is partially enclosed in deep cervical fascia. The stylomandibular ligament, a thickening of this fascia, intervenes between the parotid and submandibular glands. The outer surface of the superficial part of the gland lies in contact with the submandibular fossa above, and below is crossed by the cervical branch of the facial nerve and the facial vein (see Ch. 12). The facial artery pierces the gland and emerges between it and the insertion of the medial pterygoid on the inner side of the mandible; it then curls around the lower border of the mandible to reach the face. Submandibular lymph nodes are found on the under surface of the mandible close to the gland, and may be embedded in it. The superficial part of the gland lies on the mylohyoid muscle, and the mylohyoid nerve and vessels pass to the muscle between it and the gland. The section of gland which lies behind the posterior edge of mylohyoid lies close to the wall of the pharynx, and is related to the glossopharyngeal nerve and stylohyoid ligament.

The deep part of the gland extends forwards on the surface of hyoglossus, deep to mylohyoid.

Sandwiched between it and the hyoglossus are the lingual nerve, the submandibular ganglion, the hypoglossal nerve, and the deep lingual vein, in that order from above downwards. The submandibular duct (Wharton's duct), is a thin-walled structure which emerges from the deep part of the gland. On the surface of the hyoglossus it lies between the lingual and hypoglossal nerves. It passes medially between the sublingual gland and genioglossus and opens into the floor of the mouth on a papilla at the side of the frenulum of the tongue (Fig. 11.4). During this part of its course it is crossed laterally by the lingual nerve, which

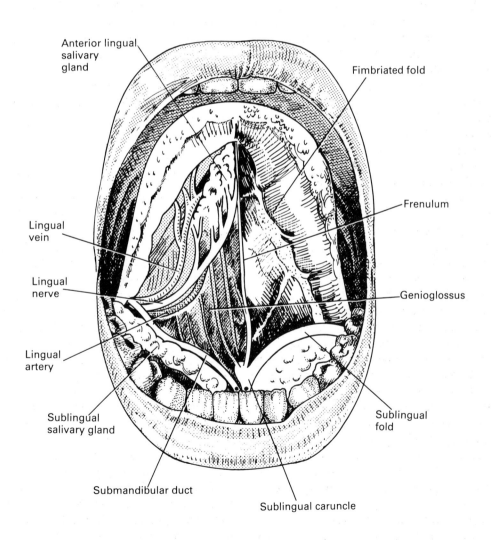

Fig. 11.4 The lingual neurovascular bundle

then ascends on the medial side of the duct, crossing it again before reaching the tongue. The close relationship of the lingual nerve to the duct must be borne in mind during surgery in the floor of the mouth. The duct can be shown on a radiogram after injection of contrast (Fig. 11.5).

The sublingual salivary gland is located beneath the floor of the mouth, close to the symphysis menti. It has about 10–20 excretory ducts which open into the floor of the mouth on the sublingual fold, or directly into the duct of the submandibular gland.

CASE 1

Prucilla Prune, a 48-year-old bus conductress, noticed a lump on the right side of her neck just below the mandible. This became painful, especially during mealtimes. The swelling subsided after a few days. She had a recurrence 2 weeks later, and sought medical advice. The swelling was in the position of the submandibular gland, and a radiograph showed the problem (Fig. 11.6). There is a large calculus in the gland. If this had been small, and located in the submandibular duct, removal would have been simple. It could have been removed through the floor of the

mouth by a small incision in the duct. Prucilla, however, had a large stone in the gland itself, and had suffered several bouts of obstructive disease. The gland was hard and tender, and it was thought best to remove it.

Operation notes

A horizontal incision was made just above the hyoid bone, extending from the sternocleidomastoid to the midline of the neck. Good exposure was required because there were several nerves closely related to the gland which needed protection. These included the marginal mandibular division of the facial nerve (see Fig. 10.15), the lingual nerve (see Fig. 11.3), and the hypoglossal nerve (see Fig. 5.5). After dividing the skin, the incision was deepened through the platysma and deep cervical fascia. The cervical fascial capsule of the gland was incised along the lower border of the gland and dissection carried out between the gland and this capsule. A flap of fascia was thus elevated towards the mandible, carrying the marginal mandibular divison of the facial nerve with it. The nerve is sometimes difficult to find, but lies well below the mandible and divides into several branches on the submandibular gland fascia. It often takes the form of several trunks. If damaged, the depressor anguli oris is paralysed, and the patient will have an asymmetrical mouth. As the gland was mobilised, the deep part was

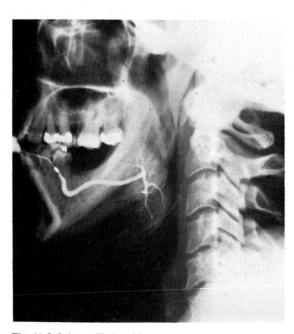

Fig. 11.5 Submandibular sialogram

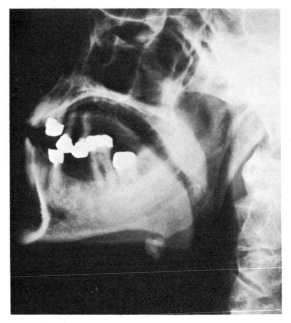

Fig. 11.6 Prucilla Prune. Radiograph of the submandibular region.

exposed by retracting the edge of the mylohyoid. During this stage, care was taken not to injure the two nerves deep to the gland, the hypoglossal and lingual nerves. The facial artery was dissected free of the gland, and the duct ligated and cut.

Prucilla made an excellent recovery. This operation went well, because it was performed by a head and neck surgeon. The student must be particularly careful when making diagnoses and prescribing surgical treatment for swellings in the submandibular region. He must never make blind incisions into abscesses, or attempt to remove deep-seated cysts, except under the best possible operative conditions. If in any doubt, a head and neck surgeon should be consulted. Damage to the nerves in the region of the gland are serious conditions, and not unknown in medicolegal circles.

CASE 2

John Studdart, a 28-year-old drug addict, presented in the emergency unit with a large, red, tender swelling of the submandibular region. He was in a bad general condition, very dirty, and had lice. His temperature was 38°. After cleaning by the nursing staff, examination of the mouth showed that he had advanced dental decay; particularly bad were the lower 2nd and 3rd molars. Radiology showed that he had a dental root abscess of the right 2nd molar tooth. He had infection of the submandibular space, a condition called 'Ludwig's angina'.

The submandibular space is bounded by the mucous membrane of the floor of the mouth above, and the deep cervical fascia that extends between the mandible and hyoid bone below. The space is partially divided by the mylohyoid, but infection spreads rapidly throughout the fascial spaces in this region. Pus rarely forms in the space, and John was treated with antibiotics. The dentist removed the lower 2nd molar tooth and drained the abscess. The swelling subsided slowly during the following few days, and when discharged, John was asked to attend for dental treatment. He failed to do so, and was seen again a few weeks later with a drug overdose.

6. The surface of the tongue

The tongue is concerned with deglutition, taste and speech. It is highly mobile, but at rest lies partly in the mouth and partly in the pharynx. The root of the tongue is attached to the hyoid bone and mandible, and is supported by the mylohyoid sling in the floor of the mouth. The surface of the dorsum of the tongue is divided into an anterior two-thirds and a posterior third by a sulcus terminalis. This is a V-shaped groove, the limbs of which extend from the foramen caecum in the midline to the palatoglossal arches on either side. The posterior third belongs to the pharynx and the anterior two-thirds to the mouth. Inspection of the oral part of the tongue will reveal numerous papillae. These are minute projections of epithelium whose function is apparently to increase the surface area available for contact and taste of fluid in the mouth. Taste buds cannot be seen with the naked eye, but are widely distributed over the surfaces of the tongue, lingual surface of the soft palate, and epiglottis. The most obvious of the papillae are the vallate papillae. These form a row of 8–12 elevations directly in front of the sulcus terminalis. Fungiform papillae are smaller, rounded, and deep red in colour. They are seen as small projections along the sides and apex of the tongue, but are also found on the dorsum. Look for these on your tongue with the aid of a magnifying glass. Filiform papillae are small, and arranged in rows parallel with the sulcus terminalis. Papillae simplices, similar to the papillae of the dermis of the skin, are found on all the surfaces of the tongue. Several elevations occur behind the sulcus terminalis on the pharyngeal part of the tongue. They are collectively called the 'lingual tonsil', and are produced by underlying lymphoid tissue. On each border of the tongue, close to the palatoglossal arch, are several vertical folds of mucous membrane called the 'foliate papillae'. The most obvious structure on the under-surface of the tongue is the frenulum. The frenulum is all that remains of the attachment of the tongue to the floor of the mouth. Occasionally ankyloglossia or tongue-tie occurs, and the tongue remains tethered to the floor. The deep lingual vein may also be seen travelling from the apex of the tongue on each side of the frenulum. Lateral to each vein is a fold of mucous membrane called the 'plica fimbriata'.

7. Development of the tongue and nerve supply

The floor of the primitive pharynx presents two lateral lingual swellings and a medial swelling called the 'tuberculum impar'. All three swellings belong to the 1st branchial arch. Behind these 1st arch structures is a median hypobranchial eminence (copula of His), formed by 2nd and 3rd branchial arch mesoderm, and some mesoderm of the 4th branchial arch. Further back is a swelling destined to become the epiglottis. The lateral lingual swellings grow rapidly and overgrow the tuberculum impar to form the anterior two-thirds of the tongue. The 2nd arch is overgrown by the 3rd arch to form the posterior third of the tongue. The foramen caecum marks the point of fusion of the constituent parts of the tongue and is also the point of downgrowth of the primitive thyroid gland. With these embryological facts in mind, the sensory nerve supply is easy to understand. The lingual branch of the mandibular nerve supplies ordinary sensation to the anterior part of the tongue in front of the sulcus terminalis. The mandibular nerve is the nerve of the 1st branchial arch. The 7th nerve, the nerve of the 2nd arch, supplies no sensation on the tongue, but its chorda tympani carries taste fibres from the taste buds *in front of* the row of vallate papillae. The glosso-

pharyngeal nerve, the nerve of the 3rd arch, supplies ordinary sensation and taste to the posterior third of the tongue, including the vallate papillae. The superior laryngeal nerve supplies sensation to the tongue immediately in front of the epiglottis. This is the nerve of the 4th arch. Occipital myotomes migrate around the pharynx into the tongue during the second month of intrauterine life, accompanied by their nerve. The hypoglossal nerve therefore supplies the musculature of the tongue.

THE ROOF OF THE MOUTH

The roof of the mouth is formed by the palate. In front this consists of the 'hard', or 'bony' palate, and behind the 'muscular', or 'soft' palate.

1. The hard palate

The bony palate is formed by the palatine processes of the maxillae and the horizontal plates of the palatine bones (Fig. 11.7). These bones are

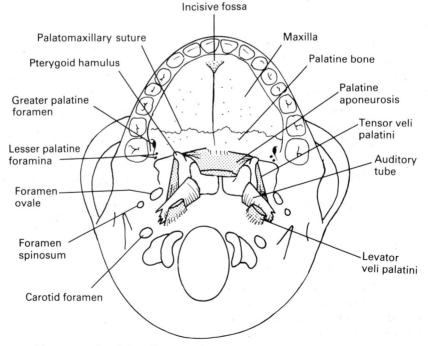

Incisive fossa

Palatomaxillary suture

Pterygoid hamulus

Maxilla

Palatine bone

Greater palatine foramen

Palatine aponeurosis

Tensor veli palatini

Lesser palatine foramina

Foramen ovale

Auditory tube

Foramen spinosum

Levator veli palatini

Carotid foramen

Fig. 11.7 The tensor and levator muscles of the palate

united at intermaxillary, interpalatine and palato-maxillary sutures. In the maxilla, behind the incisor teeth, is an incisive fossa. Two lateral incisive foramina usually lead from this fossa into canals and thence to the floor of the nose. They transmit branches of the greater palatine vessels which *ascend* into the nasal cavity, and the termination of the nasopalatine nerves, which *descend* from the nasal cavity. Occasionally, median incisive foramina will be found, and then the left nasopalatine nerve passes through the anterior and the right through the posterior median foramen. Grooves left by united sutures are often found in the region of the incisive fossa. Such a suture line can be found at birth diverging on either side from the incisive fossa to the region of the future gap between the lateral incisor and canine teeth, and may persist for several decades. Occasionally a groove is also found in the floor of the nose. It has been claimed that the maxilla in front of this line develops from two separate ossification centres and represents the premaxilla or os incisivum found in other mammals. One ossification centre has been described as being behind the incisor teeth, and the other close to the base of the nasal septum. Such a picture of ossification centres has not been confirmed, and it seems more likely that the maxilla develops from a single centre, ossifying in mesenchymal tissue. In the adult the alveolar arch contains 16 sockets for the teeth. The horizontal plates of the palatine bone end posteriorly in the midline as the posterior nasal spine. Laterally, greater and lesser palatine foramina open on the surface of the palate, and transmit palatine nerves from the pterygopalatine ganglion. A palatine crest arches medially from the greater palatine foramen. The posterolateral corner of the palatine bone is wedged in a notch between the bases of the two pterygoid plates, this projection of bone being called the 'pyramidal process of the palatine bone'.

2. The soft palate

The soft palate is a muscular fold attached to the posterior border of the hard palate. It hangs between the oral and nasal parts of the pharynx, and ends in a small conical process called the 'uvula'. Collections of lymphoid tissue and mucous glands are found beneath the mucous membrane on both surfaces of the palate. Taste buds are also found on the oral surface of the palate.

The muscle which gives the soft palate its aponeurotic support is the *tensor veli palatini*. It lies outside the pharynx, lateral to the medial pterygoid plate and the auditory tube (Fig. 11.7). It arises from the scaphoid fossa of the pterygoid process, the cartilaginous auditory tube and the spine of the sphenoid (Fig. 11.8). It gives rise to a tendon which hooks around the pterygoid hamulus, and enters the pharynx. Here it expands to form the *palatine aponeurosis*. This is attached to the posterior border of the hard palate and to the under-surface of the palate behind the palatine crest. The *levator veli palatini* arises within the pharynx from the medial and underside of the cartilaginous auditory tube. Its bony origin is from the petrous temporal bone just in front of the carotid foramen. The internal carotid artery lies close to the upper border of the superior constrictor of the pharynx outside the fossa of

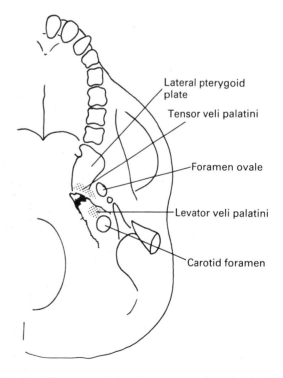

Lateral pterygoid plate

Tensor veli palatini

Foramen ovale

Levator veli palatini

Carotid foramen

Fig. 11.8 The origins of the palatine muscles from the skull

Rosenmüller, and some fibres of levator veli palatini arise from the carotid sheath in this region. The muscle inserts into the upper surface of the palatine aponeurosis, and blends with the insertion of the opposite muscle. Muscles arise from the palatine aponeurosis and descend to the tongue and pharynx. The *palatoglossus* arises from the under-surface of the aponeurosis and its fibres pass in front of the tonsil and enter the side of the tongue. The *palatopharyngeus*, a larger muscle, arises by means of two fasciculi from the upper surface of the palatine aponeurosis, the origins being separated by the insertion of levator veli palatini. Some of the fibres of the anterior fasciculus arise from the hard palate itself. The muscle descends, close to the stylopharyngeus, to gain insertion into the thyroid cartilage. The latter two muscles raise palatoglossal and palatopharyngeal folds in front of and behind the tonsillar cleft. The *palatopharyngeal sphincter*, a band of fibres arising from the upper surface of the palate and the palatine aponeurosis, sweeps around the inner surface of the superior constrictor. It raises a ridge on the inner surface of the pharynx called the 'ridge of Passavant' (see Ch. 7). The small *musculus uvulae* arises from the posterior nasal spine and inserts into the mucous membrane of the uvula. The palatine aponeurosis splits to enclose the muscle.

In the normal resting position, the oral surface of the palate is concave. The tensor palatini muscles, acting together, put tension on the palate, depress it and flatten out its arch. Acting alone, one tensor muscle will pull the soft palate to its own side. Levator veli palatini, as its name implies, is an elevator of the palate. The palatoglossus muscles can elevate the root of the tongue, but a more important function is to bring the palatoglossal arches together, and close off the mouth from the oral part of the pharynx. Palatopharyngeus pulls up the pharynx, shortening it, and assists in elevation of the larynx. During this action, the two palatopharyngeal arches approximate.

The muscles of the soft palate, with the exception of tensor veli palatini, are supplied by the cranial fibres of the accessory nerve. These reach the muscles through the pharyngeal plexus (see Ch. 7). Tensor veli palatini receives its supply from the mandibular branch of the trigeminal nerve (see Ch. 10). The sensory nerve supply to the palate is derived from branches of the pterygopalatine ganglion (palatine and nasopalatine nerves), and from the glossopharyngeal nerve. Taste fibres from the oral surface of the soft palate pass back in the lesser palatine nerve, synapse in the pterygopalatine ganglion, and reach the facial nerve in the greater petrosal nerve. They have their cell bodies in the genicular ganglion.

The arterial supply to the palate comes from three sources — the palatine branch of the ascending pharyngeal artery, the ascending palatine branch of the facial artery, and the greater palatine branch of the maxillary artery.

3. Developmental clefts of the palate

In the early embryo several swellings are apparent in the region of the future nose and mouth. Maxillary swellings are located on either side of the stomodeum, and medial and lateral nasal swellings surround the nasal pits (Fig. 11.9A). These pits are at first far apart, and the medial nasal swellings are separated in the midline by a frontal prominence. This is formed by a proliferation of mesenchyme ventral to the developing brain vesicles. As the maxillary processes continue to grow, however, the medial nasal swellings move towards the midline, meet, fuse, and overgrow the frontal process (Fig. 11.9B). The fused nasal processes are now called the 'intermaxillary segment', and on each side the maxillary swellings fuse with this segment. The intermaxillary segment is destined to form the philtrum of the upper lip, and the small segment of the palate which will carry the four incisor teeth (Fig. 11.9C). This segment of the primitive palate is continuous with the thick nasal septum formed from the frontal prominence (Fig. 11.10). At first, this broad septum is in contact with the dorsum of the developing tongue, and except for the region of the primitive palate, the nasal and oral cavities communicate with each other. During the sixth week, however, a shelf-like palatine process grows towards the midline from each maxillary swelling. At first these are separated by the tongue, but with the growth of the mandibular processes this is carried ventrally so that the palatine processes meet each other in the midline.

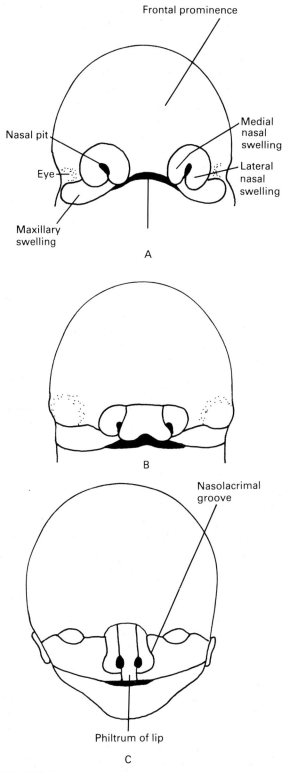

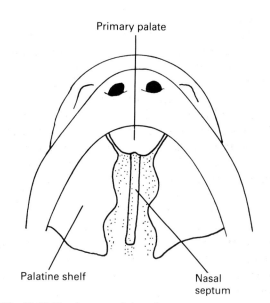

Fig. 11.10 Development of the palate

Fig. 11.9 Development of the face

Mesenchyme proliferates at the junction and the epithelial cleft between them is thus obliterated. In front, maxillary mesenchyme invades the primitive palate to bury the premaxillary segment. The only communication left between the nasal and oral cavities is found at the junction of the fused maxillary processes and the primitive palate as the nasopalatine canal. The dorsal extremities of the palatine processes fuse together to form the soft palate. 3rd branchial arch mesenchyme migrates into the position of the future palatopharyngeal folds.

Failure of fusion of the various components of the face and palate results in clefts. Of these, cleft lip and cleft palate are the common types. If one maxillary swelling fails to fuse with the intermaxillary segment, a cleft is left in the upper lip. It should be noted that such a cleft is *not* in the midline, but to one side of it. On rare occasions a midline cleft does occur, apparently because of failure of fusion of the medial nasal processes, and is then referred to as a 'hare' lip. The hare has a midline cleft in its upper lip. A more severe type of fusion failure will result in the cleft lip being continuous with a cleft between the premaxillary segment and rest of the palate (Fig. 11.11A). Bilateral cleft lip and anterior cleft palate is an ugly deformity, the clefts lying on either side of a bulbous intermaxillary segment (Fig. 11.11B). Failure of fusion of the palatine processes of the maxillary swellings results in a cleft palate behind the incisive foramen. Sometimes a complete cleft of the lip, premaxillary region, and palate occurs (Fig. 11.11C). Cleft lip is seen in about 1 in 1000 births, and is found more frequently in males than in females. The frequency of cleft palate is lower than this, occurring in about 1 in 2500 births. It is seen more often in females than in males. The main aetiological factor in the production of cleft lip and cleft palate is genetic in nature, but there is evidence that environmental factors also play a part. Drugs such as phenobarbitone and diphenylhydantoin given during pregnancy increase the risk of clefts in the fetus. Failure of the maxillary segment to merge with the lateral nasal swelling results in an oblique facial cleft, from the side of the nose to the upper lip. The nasolacrimal duct is usually exposed in such a cleft.

DEGLUTITION

The first stage of swallowing is voluntary. The tip and front of the tongue are pressed against the hard palate and the bolus of food pushed towards the back of the mouth. The soft palate descends towards the tongue, and so helps to form the bolus. The hyoid bone ascends and is fixed in this raised position by the suprahyoid and infrahyoid muscles. Elevation of the back of the tongue then pushes the bolus through the pharyngeal isthmus into the pharynx.

The second stage of swallowing is mostly involuntary. The soft palate is elevated and approximated to the posterior pharyngeal wall by contraction of the palatine musculature and the palatopharyngeal sphincter. The larynx is raised, carrying the epiglottis upwards and forwards to be squeezed between the base of the tongue and the laryngeal inlet. The epiglottis, however, is not essential in man for closure of the laryngeal inlet, and its excision does not necessarily lead to aspiration of food. The aryepiglottic folds themselves prevent food and fluid from entering the larynx.

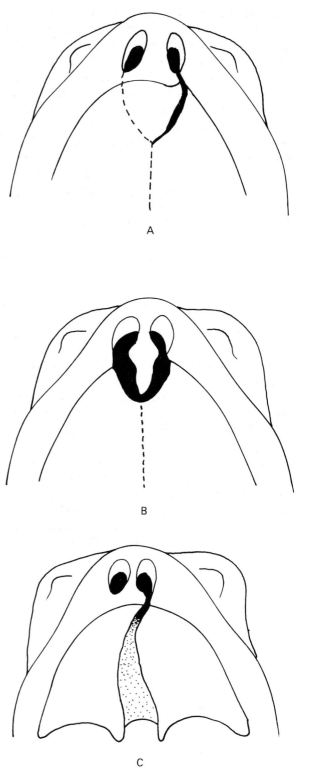

Fig. 11.11 Clefts of the lip and palate

The folds are approximated by the muscles of the laryngeal inlet, while the posterior cricoarytenoid muscles contract, pull the arytenoids back, and add to the tension in the folds. The tense folds direct food from the side of the epiglottis into lateral channels along the piriform fossae to the pharynx. Contraction of the superior and middle constrictors, together with the effect of gravity, propels the bolus to the lower pharynx. This movement is aided by the palatopharyngeus which raises the pharynx over the bolus. The third stage of deglutition takes place in the lower pharynx by contraction of the inferior constrictor, which propels the bolus into the oesophagus.

THE TEETH

In early vertebrates the dentition consists of simple conical teeth of similar shape, and there are many successions of such teeth during the lifetime of the animal. Mammals have specialised forms of teeth in different parts of the mouth (heterodont dentition), and succession is limited to two dentitions — deciduous and permanent. In man, there are five deciduous teeth in each quadrant, consisting of two incisors, one canine and two molars. There are eight permanent teeth in each quadrant — two incisors, one canine, two premolars and three molars. Details of dental morphology, histology and development are outside the scope of this text, and the student should consult a textbook of special dental anatomy for these subjects. The student of medicine, however, should have an idea of the times of dental eruption. Five tooth buds occupy each quadrant of the young jaws, and during development these migrate apart. Soon after root formation starts, the teeth move from their position in the crypts to the surface of the gum. The times of eruption of the teeth vary considerably, but the usual times of eruption of the deciduous set are as follows:

Central incisors	6–8 months
Lateral incisors	8–10 months
1st molars	12–16 months
Canines	16–20 months
2nd molars	20–30 months.

The permanent incisors and canines develop lingual to their predecessors. The permanent premolars lie deep to the deciduous molars, clasped by their divergent roots. The first permanent tooth to erupt in each quadrant is the 1st molar at 6 years of age. Soon after this the central incisor erupts, followed in sequence by the lateral incisor, canine, 1st and 2nd premolars, and 2nd molars. These have all erupted by about the age of 12 years. The 3rd molar erupts at any time between 17 and 21 years of age.

Lymph vessels from the gums pass to the submandibular nodes. Lymphatics from the floor of the mouth drain into the submental nodes and upper deep cervical nodes in front, and into the submandibular nodes further back. Lymph from the palate drains into the submandibular, upper deep cervical and retropharyngeal nodes. Lymph from the teeth drain into submandibular and deep cervical nodes.

12

THE FACE AND SCALP

THE MUSCLES OF FACIAL EXPRESSION

Although the superficial muscles of the face, the buccinator, and the platysma are usually described as the muscles of 'facial expression', they have other functions. They surround the orifices of the ear, eye, nose, and mouth, where they act as dilators and constrictors (Fig. 12.1). Loss of function of the facial muscles frequently occurs after a cerebrovascular accident, but can also follow surgical or accidental damage to the facial nerve, from which they all gain their nerve supply. Bell's palsy, possibly an inflammatory condition affecting the facial nerve, also presents with paralysis of these muscles. Loss of function is a serious problem when it limits movements of the eyelids and mouth. Of the facial muscles, therefore, the medical student should pay special attention to the musculature surrounding the eye and mouth.

1. Muscles involved in closing and opening the eye

The *orbicularis oculi* is one of the most important of the facial muscles, for if paralysed, the movement of blinking is lost. The circulation of lacrimal fluid is thus disturbed, and corneal drying and damage results. The muscle consists of three parts. The orbital part is the most peripheral of the bundles, and arises from the frontal bone and the frontal process of the maxilla at the medial side of the orbit. It also gains origin, however, from the medial palpebral ligament. Its fibres sweep widely around the eye in complete ellipses. The palpebral part of the muscle is found in the eyelids, in front

of the orbital septum. It arises from the medial palpebral ligament and adjacent bone, and its fibres sweep laterally into the upper and lower lids and intermingle at a lateral palpebral raphe. The lacrimal part of the muscle arises *behind* the lacrimal sac from the posterior crest on the lacrimal bone. Its fibres pass across the front of the tarsi to interdigitate at the lateral palpebral raphe. Some fibres enter the eyelids and insert into the tarsi close to the lacrimal canaliculi. The lacrimal part of the muscle draws the eyelids and lacrimal papillae medially, and exerting traction on the lacrimal fascia it dilates the lacrimal sac. The orbital part of the muscle is usually under voluntary control. The palpebral part can act under voluntary control, but also contracts reflexly to gently close the eyes during the act of blinking and during sleep.

The principal antagonist to the orbicularis oculi is the *levator palpebrae superioris*, an orbital muscle described in Chapter 3. The *occipitofrontalis* can also be thought of as an antagonist, for it is able to raise the eyebrows and draw the scalp backwards. It forms a broad sheet of muscle and aponeurosis over the dome of the skull. It consists of four muscle bellies — two occipital and two frontal — united by an epicranial aponeurosis (galea aponeurotica). The occipital part of the muscle gains origin from the highest nuchal line at the back of the skull. The frontal part has no bony attachment, but arises from superficial fascia and skin of the upper eyebrow, where many fibres blend with those of orbicularis oculi and other small muscles at the root of the nose. On each side, the aponeurosis is continued into the temple to gain

170

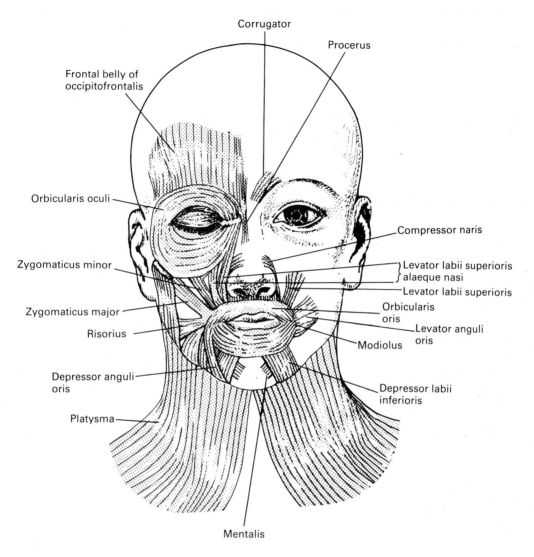

Fig. 12.1 The facial muscles

attachment to the zygomatic arch. The subcutaneous tissue of the scalp contains dense fibrous septa which unite skin to epicranial aponeurosis. Skin, subcutaneous tissue and aponeurosis should therefore be thought of as one layer. Scalp wounds that do not involve the aponeurosis do not gape, whereas those in which the aponeurosis is lacerated open widely. Wounds involving the skin, subcutaneous and aponeurotic layers bleed freely, because the blood vessels do not constrict and retract after laceration. The scalp (skin, subcutaneous tissue and aponeurosis) can be moved on the periosteum of the vault because there is a layer of loose areolar tissue deep to the aponeurosis. There is thus a potential space deep to the aponeurosis, closed posteriorly at the highest nuchal line, but open in front. Bleeding in this loose connective tissue following a head injury, tracks downwards under the influence of gravity into the upper eyelids during the first few days following the injury. The *corrugator supercillii* is a small muscle at the medial end of the eyebrow, deep to the frontal part of occipitofrontalis. Its action is to draw the eyebrow medially and downwards, a movement used during frowning.

2. Muscles of the nose

Several muscles are concerned with widening and compressing the nasal apertures during emotion and deep respiration. They are shown in Figure 12.1, but the details of their origins and insertions need not be learned by the student.

3. The muscles of the mouth

The mouth is surrounded by a considerable amount of musculature, reflecting the complexity of movements involved in mastication, speech and facial expression. The musculature consists of the sphincters (buccinator, and orbicularis oris) and the dilators (elevators, depressors and retractors). The *buccinator* arises from the outer surfaces of the alveolar processes of both maxilla and mandible, opposite the molar teeth (Fig. 12.2). Between these two origins, it arises from the pterygomandibular raphe. This structure, described in Chapter 7, extends from the pterygoid hamulus to the posterior end of the mylohyoid line of the mandible. The fibres of the buccinator converge near the angle of the mouth, where many of the middle fibres decussate and mingle with the fibres of the orbicularis oris. The uppermost fibres pass into the upper lip and the lowermost into the lower lip. Several other facial muscles also enter this decussation near the angle of the mouth, so forming a fibrous nodule called the 'modiolus'. This fibrous centre is mobile, but can be fixed by the action of muscle antagonists. The buccinator is pierced by the parotid duct opposite the upper 2nd molar tooth. The buccinator compresses the cheeks against the teeth, so that food is squeezed from the cheek pouch between the teeth. The muscles are also used during the act of blowing or whistling.

The *orbicularis oris* is made up of many layers of muscle fibres lying in several directions. Many surrounding muscles, especially the buccinator, contribute fibres to the orbicularis oris. Fibres of the incisivus labii superioris arise from the maxilla and arch into the upper lip, while the incisivus labii inferioris arises from the mandible and passes to the lower lip. Within the lips themselves, the fibres are found both within the margins and more peripherally. Many fibres lie obliquely, passing from the deep surface of the skin, through the thickness of the lip, to the mucous membrane. The actions of orbicularis oris are complicated. Apart from its use in closing the lips, it can also alter the shape of the lips. It can compress the lips against the teeth, and its decussating fibres assist in protruding the lips.

The antagonists of the sphincter muscles are elevators and retractors of the upper lip and depressors and retractors of the lower lip. The names of most of these muscles accurately describe their functions. The *levator labii superioris alaeque nasi*, arising from the maxilla, raises and everts the upper lip and assists in dilating the nostril. The *levator labii superioris* arises from the infraorbital margin, and elevates the upper lip. The *zygomaticus minor and major* arise from the zygomatic bone, and also elevate and retract the angle of the mouth laterally, a movement seen in laughing. The *levator anguli oris* arises from the maxilla just above the canine tooth, and as its name implies, raises the angle of the mouth. The *risorius* has no bony origin, but springs from the parotid fascia. It inserts into the angle of the mouth and, like the zygomatic muscles, retracts the angle of the mouth. The *depressor labii inferioris* arises from the mandible between the symphysis menti and the mental foramen, and draws the lower lip downwards. The *depressor anguli oris* also arises from the mandible and converges on the angle of the mouth, and draws the angle of the mouth downwards and laterally. The *mentalis* is a small muscle arising from the mandible below the incisor teeth. It is attached to the skin of the chin, and apart from wrinkling this skin, it helps to protrude the lower lip.

THE FACIAL NERVE

The intrapetrous course of the facial nerve is described in Chapter 4. The nerve leaves the skull through the stylomastoid foramen and enters the face. On leaving the foramen, it gives posterior auricular, digastric and stylohyoid branches. The posterior auricular nerve supplies the small auricularis posterior muscle and the occipital belly of

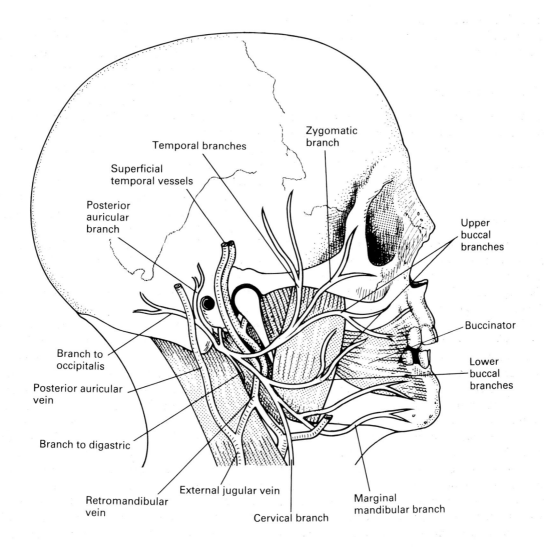

Fig. 12.2 The facial nerve

occipitofrontalis, the digastric branch the posterior belly of the digastric, and the stylohyoid branch enters the middle of that muscle. The facial nerve lies in very close proximity to the parotid gland after emerging from the stylomastoid foramen, and its course takes it into the substance of the gland. Here it divides into branches which lie superficial to both the retromandibular vein and the external carotid artery. The branches, often plexiform within the parotid, emerge from the anteromedial surface of the gland, and diverge on the face and neck to the muscles of facial expression. Although there are five named branches, there are frequent communications between the branches themselves and between them and the sensory branches of the trigeminal nerve on the face. The posterior auricular nerve often communicates with the auricular branch of the vagus, and the nerve to the digastric with the glossopharyngeal nerve. Identification, therefore, of the branches of the facial nerve during parotid surgery is by no means a simple matter. The terminal divisions of the facial nerve are described as 'temporal', 'zygomatic', 'buccal', 'marginal mandibular' and 'cervical' branches. The temporal branches cross the zygomatic arch, and supply the small muscle on the front of the auricle, and then the orbicularis oculi and the frontal belly of occipitofrontalis. Zygomatic branches cross the zygomatic bone, reach the lateral angle of the eye, and also supply the orbicularis oculi. Buccal branches have a more horizontal course, and after supplying some of the small superficial muscles around the nose, the upper branches form an infraorbital plexus with branches of the infraorbital nerve. This supplies the elevators and retractors of the upper lip. The lower branches supply the buccinator, but also send fibres to the orbicularis oris. The marginal mandibular branch is of considerable importance to the surgeon when operating in the parotid and submandibular regions. After leaving the parotid gland, it runs *below* the angle of the mandible, deep to platysma. It turns upwards over the body of the mandible and supplies the muscles of the lower lip, orbicularis oris, and risorius. If injured, therefore, functioning of that side of the mouth is severely affected. The cervical branch of the facial nerve emerges from the lower part of the parotid gland and supplies the platysma in the neck.

CASE 1 (CONTINUED FROM CHAPTER 10, CASE 3)

Adolph Hall had a parotid tumour. The mass was not large, and therefore a total conservative parotidectomy was considered. The parotid gland is removed during this procedure, but the branches of the facial nerve are left intact.

Operation notes
A vertical skin incision was made in front of the ear, extending into the upper neck. The wound was deepened until the sternocleidomastoid was exposed. The great auricular nerve was found on the surface of the muscle, and was severed. This was inevitable during the operation because its course interfered with dissection of the parotid. Postoperatively there would be a large area of anaesthesia, but this tends to shrink with the passage of time. Occasionally, a neuroma develops at the cut end of the nerve, and results in distressing pain, but such a neuroma can be destroyed by a local injection of alcohol.

The parotid dissection was started posteriorly. The sternocleidomastoid was retracted, and the posterior belly of the digastric exposed (Fig. 12.3). The facial nerve lies 4 mm deep to the cleft between the mastoid process and the bony external acoustic meatus. From here, the main trunk descends to lie above and parallel with the upper border of the posterior belly of the digastric. This part of the facial nerve was exposed carefully, so that there would be no damage to the blood supply of the nerve. The rest of the dissection traced the facial nerve branches through the substance of the parotid gland. A facial nerve stimulator was used to test the position of the branches before each step in dissection. Great care was taken in preserving the temporal and zygomatic branches because these supply the orbicularis oculi. The marginal mandibular branch of nerve was found as it left the tail of the gland. The parotid, together with the small tumour, was freed from the facial nerve branches and removed.

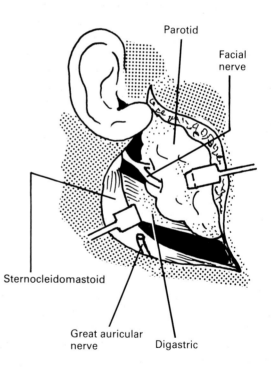

Fig. 12.3 Adolph Hall. Parotidectomy.

Postoperatively, Adolph made a good recovery, but some time later complained of discomfort, sweating and redness of the skin over the parotid area during eating. This condition, known as

'Frey's syndrome', is caused by the severed ends of parasympathetic secretomotor fibres for the parotid growing into the skin. Here they innervate blood vessels and sweat glands. An operation has been devised, using a dissecting microscope, in which the middle ear cavity is exposed and the tympanic branch of the glossopharyngeal nerve (Jacobson's nerve) sectioned. This is a fairly major procedure, however, and was not felt to be appropriate for Adolph. He was treated conservatively with applications of antiperspirant solution.

The facial nerve can be involved in Bell's palsy. This is probably a viral infection, but essentially the nerve is compressed within its facial canal. Most cases respond well to treatment, and have no residual facial weakness. In a few cases the patient is left with a facial palsy. Several plastic operations are available to raise the lower eyelid, and the corner of the mouth. The hypoglossal nerve or accessory nerve can be sectioned and anastomosed to the facial nerve. The hypoglossal nerve is usually used in preference to the accessory nerve because there is less deformity from a unilateral 12th nerve palsy than an 11th nerve palsy. Great care must be exercised during treatment of any wound situated in front of the ear. Cysts and swelling in the area should only be approached by a competent surgeon under good operating conditions.

THE FACIAL, SUPERFICIAL TEMPORAL, POSTERIOR AURICULAR, AND OCCIPITAL ARTERIES

The *facial artery* arises from the external carotid above the greater cornu of the hyoid bone. The artery grooves the posterior border of the submandibular gland or actually pierces it. It emerges between the gland and the medial pterygoid insertion, hooks around the lower border of the mandible and enters the face. In the living state its pulsations may be palpated in this part of its course. On the face it takes an oblique course, past the angle of the mouth, deep to the zygomaticus major, and then proceeds to its termination at the medial palpebral commissure. Here, it anastomoses with terminal branches of the ophthalmic artery. The ascending palatine and tonsillar branches of the facial artery arise in the neck, and are described in Chapter 7. As it traverses the submandibular gland, the facial artery gives branches to the gland and a submental artery to the chin and lower lip. In its facial course, the artery gives superior and inferior labial branches. The superior of these gives a septal branch which ramifies on the lower and anterior part of the nasal septum. Here it anastomoses with terminal branches of the sphenopalatine artery in Little's area, and it is in this region that an epistaxis commonly occurs.

The *superficial temporal artery* is the smaller of the two terminal branches of the external carotid. It begins within the substance of the parotid gland, behind the neck of the mandible. Here it gives a branch called the 'transverse facial artery', which travels forwards between the parotid duct and the zygomatic arch (see Fig. 10.15). It anastomoses with branches of the facial artery. The main trunk of the superficial temporal artery crosses the zygoma, and its pulsations can be palpated just above the zygomatic arch, in front of the ear. This is a convenient place for an anaesthetist to take the pulse of a patient. The artery gives branches to the ear, and a zygomatico-orbital branch which continues along the upper border of the zygomatic arch to anastomose with terminal branches of the ophthalmic artery. The superficial temporal artery, after giving these branches, divides into anterior, middle and posterior temporal branches. The anterior branch of the superficial temporal artery (external carotid) can establish anastomoses with the supraorbital artery (internal carotid) in the scalp. The *occipital and posterior auricular arteries* are branches of the external carotid, and lie in close relationship to the posterior belly of the digastric. The occipital artery is overlapped by the inferior border of the digastric, and at its origin is crossed superficially by the hypoglossal nerve. The artery gives branches to the sternocleidomastoid, the mastoid process, mastoid air cells, and ends by supplying suboccipital muscles and scalp. The posterior auricular artery runs along the upper border of the digastric and stylohyoid. It gives branches to the auricle and the occipital region. It gives a stylomastoid artery which enters the foramen of the same name, and supplies the tympanic cavity and mastoid antrum.

Incisions in the scalp must take account of the

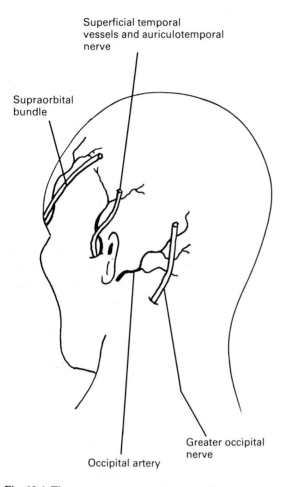

Fig. 12.4 The cutaneous nerves and vessels of the scalp

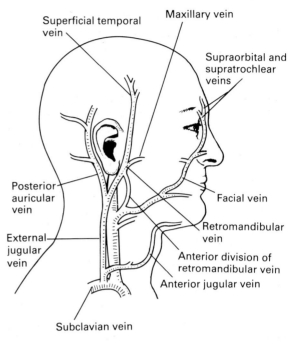

Fig. 12.5 The veins of the head and neck

positions of cutaneous nerves and vessels (Fig. 12.4). In front, care must be exercised with the supraorbital neurovascular bundle, and at the side, with the auriculotemporal nerve and superficial temporal artery. At the back of the skull, the occipital artery and greater occipital nerve should be avoided.

SUPERFICIAL VEINS OF THE FACE AND NECK (Fig. 12.5)

The *facial vein* is formed by the union of supraorbital and supratrochlear veins. It passes obliquely down the face, following a course similar to the facial artery. This takes it past the nose, under cover of zygomaticus major, past the angle of the mouth to the body of the mandible. Below the mandible it lies superficial to the submandibular gland, and is joined by the anterior division of the retromandibular vein. Its course is then superficial to the loop of the lingual artery and the hypoglossal nerve. It ends by joining the internal jugular vein. The facial vein communicates with the cavernous sinus near the medial side of the orbit through connections between it and the ophthalmic veins. The facial vein has no valves, and superficial infections of the lower face can spread along the facial vein to the cavernous sinus, causing a cavernous sinus infection and thrombosis. This condition is fortunately rarely seen nowadays, for when it occurs it is usually fatal. In pre-antibiotic days, cases were seen from time to time, and the area of the face from the side of the nose to the angle of the mouth was designated the 'dangerous area' of the face because it was in this region that infection could lead to cavernous sinus thrombosis. Another communication between the facial vein and the cavernous sinus takes place via a large plexus of veins around the pterygoid muscles. Input into the pterygoid plexus from the cavernous sinus arrives in veins which pass either through the foramen ovale, foramen lacerum, or a foramen of Vesalius. The pterygoid plexus drains into the facial vein through a short vessel, the deep facial vein.

Much of the blood from the pterygoid plexus of veins leaves in the *maxillary vein*. The vein joins the *superficial temporal vein* within the parotid gland to form the *retromandibular vein*. This vein lies deep to the facial nerve and superficial to the external carotid artery within the substance of the gland. As it descends through the gland, it forms two divisions. The anterior division joins the facial vein, and the posterior division unites with the *posterior auricular vein* to form the *external jugular vein*. This latter vessel descends on the sterno-cleidomastoid muscle, and just above the middle of the clavicle perforates the deep cervical fascia and enters the subclavian vein. It has two pairs of valves near its termination. The external jugular vein is occasionally used for central venous can-nulation, but its size is variable, and it is often difficult to manipulate the cannula through the lower part of the vein. The *posterior external jugular vein* drains blood from the occipital region and en-ters the external jugular on the sternocleidomastoid. Veins from the submandibular region form an *an-terior jugular vein* near the hyoid bone. This vessel descends in front of the strap muscles and then turns laterally behind the sternocleidomastoid and enters the subclavian vein. The anterior jugular veins are united across the midline above the manubrium by a jugular venous arch.

Scalp veins are often used in the young baby for setting up an intravenous infusion. The veins are easily seen, and can be made prominent by using a head-down position. A small needle can be in-troduced and fixed to the skin with plaster. It is a useful position, because it does not interfere with the limb movements of the child.

LYMPH DRAINAGE OF THE FACE

Lymph vessels from the eyelids drain into the parotid group of nodes. Medially, vessels from the eyelids follow the facial vein to the submandibular group of nodes. Much of the lymph from the front of the face follows the facial vessels to the submandibular nodes. There are often a few buc-cal nodes on this route at the side of the cheek. The central part of the lower lip drains to the sub-mental nodes. Lymph from the forehead and side of the face drains mainly into the parotid group of nodes.

SENSORY SUPPLY IN THE FACE AND SCALP

Figure 12.6 shows a summary of the sensory branches of trigeminal nerve. The anterior surface of the pinna is supplied by branches of the auri-culotemporal nerve (mandibular nerve) and the great auricular nerve (cervical plexus). Some skin in the meatus is supplied by the auricular branch of the vagus nerve. Skin at the back of the ear is sup-plied by the great auricular, lesser occipital, auricu-lotemporal and the auricular branch of the vagus.

MAXILLOFACIAL RADIOLOGY

Maxillofacial fractures commonly follow direct trauma to the face as a result of a fight or an ac-cident. Automobile accidents frequently result in facial trauma, especially if the victim was not wear-ing a seat-belt at the time of the accident. Facial injuries also follow accidents at work or sport, and many of these cases occur in the young adult age-group. Treatment of severe facial fractures should be undertaken by a faciomaxillary specialist. It is important, however, that the student should be able to read the standard films used in the initial assessment of faciomaxillary trauma. Special atten-tion should be paid to bony continuity in the orbit, zygomatic arches, and maxillae. Of the projections already studied, the *Caldwell's, Waters', verticosub-mental, and lateral views* are particularly suitable for initial analysis. The *Caldwell projection* is par-ticularly useful for examining the floor of the orbit, the orbital margins, and the superior orbital fis-sure. The lines of continuity to be followed around

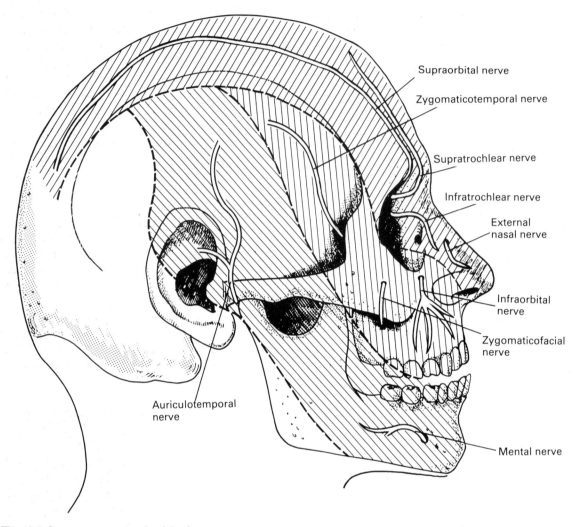

Fig. 12.6 Cutaneous nerve supply of the face

the orbit are shown in Figure 12.7. The orbital margin is first outlined, and should have no break in continuity (line A in Fig. 12.7). The student should, however, remember that the zygomatico-frontal suture is visible on the lateral orbital margin, and that the zygomaticomaxillary suture may be seen on the inferior orbital margin. When tracing the medial orbital margin, two lines are usually seen, the line within the orbital margin being made by the posterior lacrimal crest of the lacrimal bone (line B in Fig. 12.7). Within the orbit, the superior orbital fissure will be seen extending obliquely upwards from the medial orbital margin towards the centre of the orbit. The outer margin of the

frontal bone, zygoma and zygomatic arch should then be outlined (line C in Fig. 12.7). Of the midline structures, the frontal air sinuses should be closely inspected, but the view is not suitable for examination of the nasal bones, because they are seen end-on. The nasal septum can, however, be inspected. The *Waters' view* is the projection used for examination of the middle part of the face. The opportunity should be taken to inspect the lower orbital margin again (line A in Fig. 12.8). The maxillary sinuses should be examined, but these must not be confused with a large translucent area on either side bounded by the zygomatic arch, maxilla and mandible. Within this area the coron-

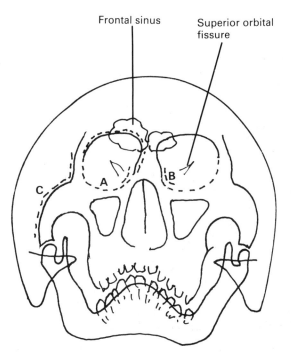

Fig. 12.7 The Caldwell projection

oid process can be seen end-on. The Waters' view is particularly useful for inspection of the zygomatic arch. One line should be traced along its inferior border (line B in Fig. 12.8), and the other along its superior border (line C is Fig. 12.8). It is said that these two lines taken together resemble the drawing of an elephant's head and trunk.

The *verticosubmental view* can be used for inspection of the profiles of the zygomatic arches (see Fig. 1.18). The relationship between the mandibular condyles and the mandibular fossae can also be established. Ethmoidal air sinuses are seen through the front of the palate in this projection, and an opacity of these sinuses usually indicates trauma and bleeding. The *lateral view* of the skull must also be taken in the initial assessment of facial injury (Fig. 12.9). Frontal and maxillary air sinuses should be inspected. The frontal bone and front end of the hard palate should lie in the same vertical plane, with the upper surface of the hard palate lying at right angles to it. The hard palate should be parallel to the lower surface of the sphenoid, and a vertical line from the sphenoidal

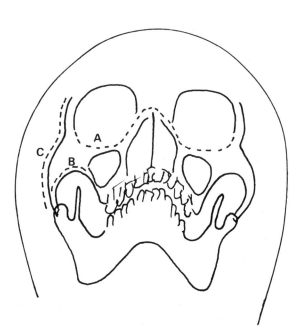

Fig. 12.8 The Waters' projection

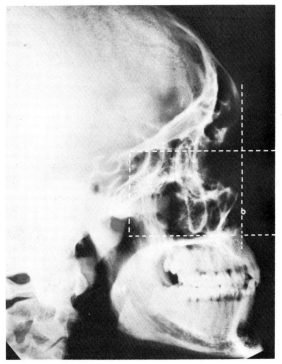

Fig. 12.9 Lateral view of the face

sinus to the back of the hard palate should be at right angles to it. Computed tomography is essential in suspected faciomaxillary injury. The signs of injury may be subtle, and therefore the soft tissues of the face must be examined for swelling and the sinuses scrutinised for opacity. Fractures involving the paranasal air sinuses sometimes lead to subcutaneous or intracranial collections of air. Facial injuries may be localised to the region of the blow, but may also involve adjacent structures. When examining a fracture of the superior orbital margin, for example, the frontal sinus must be carefully inspected to exclude extension of the fracture into the sinus wall. Fracture of the lower orbital margin can be serious, and involve the infraorbital nerve, and therefore sensation on the front of the cheek must be tested in such cases. A fragment of the lower orbital margin, together with periorbital fat, is sometimes displaced into the roof of the maxillary air sinus in an injury called a 'blow out' fracture. The support for the eyeball may thus be partially lost, and the patient complains of double vision (diplopia). When examining orbital margin fractures, the ethmoidal air sinuses should be inspected, because the ethmoid in the medial orbital wall is delicate and easily broken. An opaque ethmoidal sinus from bleeding after such a break may sometimes be the only clue to a serious orbital fracture. Fractures of the zygomatic process, zygomatic arch and nasal bones, require special views. Direct blows to the upper jaw may fracture the alveolar margin and the teeth, and such patients will be transferred for dental care. A direct blow over the malar eminence of the zygomatic bone may separate a zygomatic fragment from the frontal, temporal and maxillary attachments to produce a so-called 'tripod fracture'.

Sometimes facial injury is widespread, and fractures extend across the orbits and maxillae to produce large and complex fragments. A French investigator, Rene LeFort, defined certain lines of weakness in the facial skeleton. The first line of weakness extends across the mid-maxillae and pterygoid plates (line A in Fig. 12.10). This region

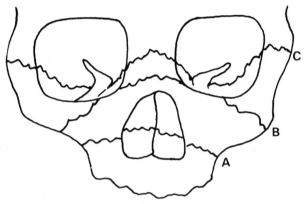

Fig. 12.10 LeFort weakness lines

is usually injured by a direct blow to the front of the face, and such an injury is called a 'LeFort I fracture'. The second type of fracture occurs across a line of weakness through the ethmoid, floor of the orbit, and the lateral wall of the maxilla, and results from a blow to the root of the nose (line B in Fig. 12.10). The third line of weakness extends across the ethmoids into the floor of the orbits, across the infraorbital fissures, and into the lateral wall of the orbit and zygomatic arches (line C in Fig. 12.10). Combinations of these fractures are frequently found.

INDEX